User Guide To Lipid Disorder Management

by

DAVID A. LEAF, M.D., M.P.H.

Assistant Professor
Division of Nutrition
Department of Medicine
University of California
Los Angeles, California

Second Edition

EMIS

Essential Medical
Information Systems, Inc.
Durant, Oklahoma

Direct Mail Orders
Essential Medical
Information Systems, Inc.
P.O. Box 1607
Durant, Oklahoma 74702-1607

Telephone Orders
1-800-225-0694

FAX Your Order
(405) 924-9414

EMIS

ISBN: 0-929240-44-8

Printed in the United States of America

Center Index Texts Published By
Essential Medical Information Systems, Inc.

Managing Contraceptive Pill Patients – 6th Ed. – *Dickey*

Emergency Cardiac Maneuvers – 2nd Ed. – *Bartecchi*

Management of Hypertension – 4th Ed. – *Kaplan*

Contraceptive Surgery For Men and Women – 2nd Ed. *Moss/AVSC*

Hormonal Contraception: ***Pills, Injections and Implants*** – *Goldzieher*

Breastfeeding: ***A Problem-Solving Manual*** – 3rd Ed. – *Saunders, Carroll & Johnson*

Management of Infertility: ***A Clinician's Manual*** – 2nd Ed. – *Cohen*

Family Planning ***At Your Fingertips*** – *Hatcher, et al*

Arthritis Therapy: ***A Clinician's Manual*** – *Kantor*

Management of Heart Failure – *Cohn & Kubo*

Menopause: ***Clinical Concepts*** – *London & Chihal*

Premenstrual Syndrome – 2nd Ed. – *Chihal*

Management of Diabetes Mellitus – 2nd Ed. – *Schwartz*

Managing Danazol Patients – 2nd Ed. – *Dickey*

Hormone Replacement Therapy – 3rd Ed. – *Grambrell*

Understanding Endometriosis – *Corson*

Call 1-800-225-0694 or FAX Your Order to: 405/924-9414

DEDICATION

This book is dedicated to my wife, Leslee, and our little daughter, Chanel, for the joy and warmth they give to my life; to Mr. Ronald James Padovana for providing a special and personal source of inspiration for the majority of my life; for my friends and colleagues; and, for the dedicated scientists whose career devotion to this important aspect of disease prevention continues to provide insights and direction in this field and contributes to our quality of living.

TABLE OF CONTENTS

TABLES

FIGURES

CENTER INDEX SYSTEMS

The purpose of the center index system is to enable readers to immediately locate all the information contained in the book. Tabs are provided with each center index so there is a direct connection between the center index and text. The text is organized in a sequential format to enable the reader to proceed to any area of the text without having to read through information not relevant to the situation.

#1 Cholesterol and Coronary Artery Disease

The Cholesterol Hypothesis

Although the cholesterol hypothesis has been subjected to longstanding debate, recent research has provided strong evidence in support of this position and has served to stimulate the formation of national guidelines aimed at lowering plasma cholesterol levels.

According to the cholesterol hypothesis, elevated levels of plasma cholesterol directly contribute to the pathogenesis of atherosclerotic disease, which ultimately causes coronary artery disease (CAD). CAD is the result of both thrombogenic and progressive atherogenic occlusion of the arterial blood vessel lumen.

Early evidence in support of the cholesterol hypothesis was derived from plaque studies and feeding experiments in primate models. Similarly, epidemiological evidence supports the direct relationship between plasma cholesterol levels and CAD risk.

In spite of these findings, only recently has more conclusive evidence been available to support the cholesterol hypothesis with the completion of prospective, randomized, double-blind, control intervention trials. These indicate that lowering of plasma cholesterol levels can reduce CAD risk and cause disease regression.

It should be recognized that "plasma cholesterol" from the perspective of the cholesterol hypothesis refers to total plasma cholesterol levels as a reflection of plasma LDL-C, the atherogenic plasma lipoprotein. Thus, plasma cholesterol values as a predictor of CAD risk are a surrogate, reflecting plasma LDL-C levels.

Recent Prospective Trials

THE LIPID RESEARCH CLINICS CORONARY PRIMARY PREVENTION TRIAL (LRC-CPPT)

This double-blind, placebo-controlled trial, randomized 3,806 asymptomatic hypercholesterolemic (Type IIa) men to receive diet (low fat, low cholesterol) intervention plus one of the following:

- Cholestyramine (Questran®)
- Placebo

After seven years of intervention, the experiments resulted in:

- The incidence of CAD events in seven percent of the cholestyramine group
- The incidence of CAD events in 8.6 percent of the placebo group
- A 19 percent reduction in CAD events in the treated group associated with the reduction in total cholesterol (13.4 percent) and LDL cholesterol (20.3 percent)
- An eight percent reduction in total cholesterol associated with a 19 percent reduction in CAD risk (one to two ratio)
- A 25 percent reduction in total plasma cholesterol levels in the men who took the full therapeutic medication dose, corresponding with a 49 percent reduction in fatal and nonfatal CAD events

THE HELSINKI HEART STUDY (THHS)

This randomized, double-blind, prospective primary prevention trial compared:

- The effects of gemfibrozil placebo on plasma lipids and lipoproteins
- Incidence of CAD events in 4,081 Finnish men (Types IIa, IIb and IV)

After five years, this study resulted in:

- A 34 percent total reduction of CAD events in the gemfibrozil group (most evident in the subgroups of men with elevated plasma triglyceride levels, Types IIb and IV)
- Reduction of CAD risk by three to five percent associated with a one percent increase in plasma HDL-C levels

THE CHOLESTEROL-LOWERING ATHEROSCLEROSIS STUDY (CLAS)

This secondary prevention, placebo-controlled study involved men who had undergone coronary artery bypass graft surgery. It was designed to assess the effect of plasma cholesterol lowering using a combination therapy of colestipol (Colestid®) and niacin with dietary intervention on angiographic findings.

Compared with the placebo group, the men receiving medication therapy experienced:

- Plasma LDL-C reduction of 43 percent
- Plasma triglyceride reduction of 22 percent
- Increase in plasma HDL-C of 37 percent
- A regression of lesions by 16 percent

These changes in plasma lipids and lipoproteins were also associated with a decrease in the number of new lesions noted in both native arteries and vein grafts. In addition, less disease progression was evident in the native vessels of the treated group.

THE FAMILIAL ATHEROSCLEROSIS TREATMENT STUDY (FATS)

This prospective 2.5 year study in hypercholesterolemic men with elevated apo-B levels and angiographically documented CAD compared the effect of random assignment to either niacin plus colestipol, lovastatin plus colestipol or less aggressive conventional therapy.

- Plasma LDL-C was reduced (paralleled by apo-B changes) by 32 percent with niacin and colestipol, 46 percent with lovastatin and colestipol and 7 percent by conventional therapy
- Greater angiographic evidence of regression was noted in the aggressive therapy groups
- Multivariate analysis showed benefit was predicted by reduced apo-B, systolic blood pressure and increased HDL-C.
- More clinical events occured in the conventional group (II), compared with lovastatin/colestipol (3), and niacin plus colestipol (2)

LIFESTYLE HEART STUDY

This prospective secondary prevention trial compared the effects of an aggressive non-pharmaceutical intervention (7 percent dietary fat, exercise and relaxation program) with a usual care (30 percent dietary fat) on angiographically documented CAD. One year of follow-up of 195 lesions showed:

- Intervention group—Mean stenosis diameter diminished from 40.0 to 37.8 percent
- Control group—Mean stenosis diameter increased from 42.7 to 46.1 percent
- Regression was greatest in the subjects with the greatest adherence score

Relationship Between Plasma Cholesterol Level and CAD Risk

Although the presence of a continuous relationship between plasma cholesterol levels and CAD has been suggested, findings from the Multiple Risk Factor Intervention Trial (MRFIT) recently confirmed the existence of this relationship. Figure 3.1 (see Section #3) shows the relationship between serum cholesterol levels in the group of 325,348 men during screening and the age-adjusted incidence of CAD-related mortality during a five-year period of subsequent follow-up.

Despite the definite direct relationship between serum cholesterol levels and CAD risk shown in these findings, this relationship is notably curvilinear. This indicates that, although lower plasma cholesterol levels represent a lower CAD risk, there appears to be an aspect of diminishing returns.

Clearly, plasma cholesterol lowering in the hypercholesterolemic is important for CAD risk reduction. This is especially exemplified by the previous clinical intervention trials, which involved hypercholesterolemic men. Similar trials have not been conducted in women and normocholesterolemics, although as discussed in Section 27 recent evidence indicates that regression can also occur in women with appropriate therapy. Although from the individual patient's standpoint, high plasma cholesterol levels bear an increased risk for CAD, it is important to recognize that in terms of population attributable risk, nearly half of CAD-related mortality occurs between the plasma cholesterol range of 190 to 249 mg% (4.9 to 6.4 mmol/L). In addition, the effect of cholesterol lowering appears to have a substantially greater impact in reducing CAD risk in those with established CAD than in the primary prevention setting.

Therefore, regarding public health, all efforts aimed at lowering the population's mean plasma cholesterol level from its current value of approximately 210 mg% (5.4 mmol/L) are beneficial measures for society as a whole.

The Importance of Plasma HDL-C Level In CAD Risk

Although international correlates of plasma HDL-C levels with CAD risk are not as predictive as is plasma LDL-C, plasma HDL-C levels show a well-established inverse relationship to CAD risk in Western cultures. The current recommendation for the treatment of hypercholesterolemia focuses on reduction of atherogenic LDL-C levels.

Although few animal studies are available involving plasma HDL-C and CAD risk, plasma HDL-C levels may explain the gender differences in CAD risk. Similarly, postmenopausal estrogen use raises plasma HDL-C levels and lowers CAD risk. Certainly, there is an appropriate pathophysiological model of the mechanism by which HDL-C can reduce atherosclerosis.

The exclusion of HDL-C from current formally-sanctioned treatment schemes also stems from the difficulty in interpretation of research studies assessing the effects of plasma HDL-C changes. Plasma HDL-C alterations do not occur in isolation and are confounded by concomitant changes in other plasma lipoprotein levels. Thus, it remains difficult to decipher the interactive effects of plasma HDL-C and LDL-C changes. Also, certain genetic disorders with low plasma HDL-C levels do not appear to cause increased CAD risk.

In addition, from the clinical standpoint, the measurement of plasma HDL-C levels is problematic. This is because lab variability in the measurement of the relatively small value of plasma HDL-C can have a proportionately greater influence on plasma HDL levels than is the case of plasma total cholesterol. Similarly, current laboratory standardization is not available for plasma HDL-C, as it is for total cholesterol, which means HDL-C measurements are less accurate in the clinical setting than are plasma LDL-C measurements.

Furthermore, few clinical measures are available that can safely promote plasma HDL-C increases. In our cost-minded health care system, the added cost/benefit ratio of plasma HDL-C levels remains to be shown.

In contrast, a growing body of epidemiological evidence continues to identify the powerful inverse relationship between plasma HDL-C levels and CAD risk. Therefore, this issue remains to be settled.

Recent findings based on the combined evaluation of four major prospective American studies indicate that a one percent increase in plasma HDL-C level is associated with a reduction in CAD risk of:

- Two percent for men
- Three percent for women

Using a proportional hazards model, the LRC-CPPT study indicated a small, but significant, CAD-lowering effect of increasing plasma HDL-C levels.

The Helsinki Heart Study found that the best benefit in CAD risk reduction gained by raising plasma HDL-C occurred for the men with plasma HDL-C levels below 35 mg% (0.9 mmol/L). Also, in the study population with the highest baseline levels of plasma LDL-C, the plasma HDL-C lipoprotein fraction provided the greatest predictive value for CAD risk. The severity of LDL-C elevation did not provide any predictive value of CAD risk.

The Framingham Study showed that even at lower cholesterol levels (below 200 mg [5.2 mmol/L]), lower plasma HDL-C levels are associated with increased rates of CAD in both men and women. Although the HDL_2-C subfraction has been generally regarded as the most protective HDL particle, growing evidence also supports the importance of the HDL_3-C subparticle.

Certainly the current guidelines are no replacement for clinical judgment. Hopefully, continued research findings will help to clarify the HDL-C issue and provide directives for more concrete clinical guidelines which incorporate HDL-C directly in the management strategies.

The Total-Cholesterol/HDL-C Ratio and CAD Risk

The concept of combining the CAD predictive capacity of plasma total cholesterol (ie, LDL-C) and plasma HDL-C levels was initially suggested by findings from the Framingham Study, which provided evidence that the total-cholesterol/HDL-C ratio was predictive of CAD risk. Although not utilized by current guidelines, the concept of this ratio should not be ignored, especially when individual CAD risk-factor management is involved.

In view of Framingham Study findings indicating that HDL-C is predictive of CAD risk in individuals with total plasma cholesterol levels below 200 mg% (5.2 mmol/L), a resurgence in the use of this index may arise and can be useful for individualizing patient care. Table 1.1 provides some total-cholesterol/HDL-C ratio standards which the clinician may find useful for individualizing current guidelines.

TABLE 1.1 – **Mean Ratios of Total Cholesterol to HDL-C in Various Populations (Framingham Heart Study)**

Group	Total Cholesterol/ HDL-C Ratio
Vegetarians	2.8
1/2 standard risk	3.4
Boston marathon runners (physicians)	3.4
Standard risk (women)	4.4
Standard risk (men)	5.0
Average victim (women)	4.6 to 6.4
Average victim (men)	5.5 to 6.1
3 x standard risk (women)	11.0
3 x standard risk (men)	23.4

References

Abbott RD, Wilson PWF, et al: High density lipoprotein cholesterol, total cholesterol screening and myocardial infarction: the Framingham study. Arteriosclerosis 1988;8:207.

Blankenhorn DH, Nessim SA, et al: Beneficial effects of combined colestipol-niacin therapy on coronary atherosclerosis and coronary venous bypass grafts (CLAS). JAMA 1987;257:3233.

Brown G, Albers JJ, Fisher LD, et al: Regression of coronary heart disease as a result of intensive lipid-lowering therapy in men with high levels of apolipoprotein B. N Engl J Med 1990;323:1289.

Castelli WP, Abbott RD, McNamara PM: Summary of estimates of cholesterol used to predict coronary heart disease. Circulation 1983;67:4.

Castelli WP, Garrison RJ, et al: Incidence of coronary heart disease and lipoprotein cholesterol levels: The Framingham study. JAMA 1986; 256:2835.

Crique MH: Cholesterol, primary and secondary prevention and all-cause mortality. Ann Intern Med 1991;115:973.

Frick MH, Elo O, et al: Helsinki Heart Study: primary prevention trial with gemfibrozil in middle-aged men with dyslipidemia. N Engl J Med 1987; 317:1237.

Gordon DJ, Probstfeld JL, et al: High-density lipoprotein cholesterol and cardiovascular disease: four prospective American studies. Circulation 1989;79:8.

Grundy SM, Goodman DWS, et al: The place of HDL in cholesterol management: a perspective from the National Cholesterol Education Program. Arch Intern Med 1989;149:505.

Kannel WB, Neaton JD, et al: Overall and CHD mortality rates in relationship to major risk factors in 325,348 men screened for the MRFIT. Am Heart J 1986;122:825.

Lipid Research Clinics Program: The Lipid Research Clinics Primary Prevention Trial results: reduction in incidence of coronary heart disease. JAMA 1984;251:351.

Marmot MG: Hypercholesterolemia: a public health problem. Atheroscler Rev 1988;18:95.

Olson RE: A critique of the report of the National Institutes of Health Expert Panel on Detection, Evaluation and Treatment of High Blood Cholesterol. Arch Intern Med 1989;1501.

Ornish D, Brown SE, Scherwitz LW, et al: Can lifestyle changes reverse coronary heart disease? Lancet 1990;336:129.

Stampfer MJ, Sacks FM, Salvinis CT, et al: A prospective study of cholesterol, apolipoproteins and the risk of myocardial infarction. N Engl J Med 1991;325:373.

Superko HR, Bachovik PS, Wood PD: High-density lipoprotein cholesterol measurements: a help or hindrance in practical clinical medicine? JAMA 1986;256:2714.

#2 Measurement of Plasma Cholesterol

2.

Cholesterol Screening

An accurate determination of plasma cholesterol level is critical for both identification and management of the dyslipidemic disorder. Every adult over the age of 20 years should be screened to determine their total plasma cholesterol level. For cholesterol screening purposes, the individual need not necessarily be in a fasted condition. However, it is best that this test be conducted no sooner than three months following an acute medical illness (including a myocardial infarction) because the metabolic influences of major disease processes can alter plasma lipid levels.

Automated or fingerstick procedures are acceptable methods for routine cholesterol screening purposes, although the reliability of lipid measurements varies between instruments even under controlled measurement conditions. The results can be used to identify individuals requiring further diagnostic testing.

Diagnostic Testing

The diagnosis of hypercholesterolemia needs to be determined from a venous blood sample drawn following a 12 to 14 hour (overnight) fast. Because of concerns involving measurement error, the Center For Disease Control has established standardization criteria for participating laboratories.

It is best to employ the services of a nationally standardized laboratory in analyzing plasma lipid and lipoprotein specimens. Current efforts are being made to improve clinical laboratory performance (accuracy and reproducibility) of total plasma cholesterol measurements in an approximate three percent range.

Besides the measurement of total plasma cholesterol levels, determination of plasma lipoproteins is important for both therapeutic and diagnostic purposes. Most laboratories use precipitation methods in determining the necessary lipid measurements required to establish the lipoprotein profile, including:

- Plasma total cholesterol
- HDL-C
- Triglyceride levels

For this purpose, the LDL-cholesterol value can be calculated from the Friedewald formula when plasma triglycerides are below 400 mg% (4.5 mmol/L):

$$\text{LDL-C} = \text{Total cholesterol} - [(\text{Triglycerides} \div 5) + \text{HDL-C}]$$

The VLDL particle triglyceride enrichment that occurs with hypertriglyceridemia alters the usual 1:5 cholesterol/triglyceride ratio when plasma triglyceride values exceed 400 mg% (4.5 mmol/L). Ultracentrifugation techniques are necessary to measure plasma VLDL-C levels accurately in these individuals. In this setting, LDL-C can be calculated by subtracting the directly measured VLDL-C and HDL-C from total cholesterol.

Ultracentrifugation (beta quantification) techniques can also be employed for the diagnosis of Type III dyslipidemia, or dysbeta-lipoproteinemia. In this condition, the VLDL-C particle undergoes relative cholesterol enrichment, causing the ratio of VLDL-C cholesterol/triglyceride to exceed three to 10 in comparison with the normal one to five relationship.

In practice, the diagnosis of this dyslipidemia is made by obtaining a fasting plasma VLDL-C value by ultracentrifugation and a simultaneous total triglyceride level. A ratio of VLDL-C/total triglycerides exceeding 0.3 is then diagnostic.

Lipoprotein electrophoresis depicts an alternative technique for establishing the Type III diagnosis. This non-quantitative technique can demonstrate the presence of the broad band ("floating") beta particle that is characteristic of this disorder.

Although not yet directly applicable for the patient management setting, specialized laboratory techniques are available for measurements of LDL-C and HDL-C subparticle fractions. Although national standardization is not developed, measurement of plasma apolipoprotein values is employed by some commercial and research laboratories.

Monitoring

A period of approximately four weeks is required in order to optimally judge the full effects of either dietary and/or pharmaceutical interventions on plasma lipid and lipoprotein values. Therefore, it is suggested that a minimum of four weeks should elapse between plasma lipid measurement determination during treatment.

An exception to this recommendation occurs in the clinical setting of severe hypertriglyceridemia (with chylomicronemia), where frequent measurements of plasma triglyceride levels are necessary to gauge the impact of urgent triglyceride-lowering therapy in clearing the chylomicronemia.

Because plasma LDL-C values and not total plasma cholesterol values form the basis of the current rationale for the management of hypercholesterolemia, a determination of fasting measurements of plasma lipids and lipoproteins is necessary in the management of lipid disorders.

References

Jacobs D, Barrett-Conner E: Re-test reliability of plasma cholesterol and triglycerides: the Lipid Research Clinic's prevalence study. Am J Epidemiol 1982;116:878.

Kaufman HW, McNamara JR, et al: How reliably can compact chemistry analyzers measure lipids? JAMA 1990;263:1245.

Frederickson DS, Morgonroth J, Levy RI: Type III hyperlipoproteinemia: an analysis of two contemporary definitions. Ann Intern Med 1975;82:150.

Friedewald W, Levy RI, Frederickson D: Estimation of the concentration of low density lipoprotein in plasma without use of the preparative ultracentrifuge. Clin Chem 1972;18:499.

Naughton MJ, Luepker RV, Strickland D: The accuracy of portable cholesterol analyzers in public health screening programs. JAMA 1990; 263:1213.

Roberts L: Measuring cholesterol is as tricky as lowering it. Science 1987;238:282.

#3 Definition of Hypercholesterolemia

Definition by Cholesterol Levels

A clear definition of what constitutes hypercholesterolemia is not established. The cutoff criteria used to define hypercholesterolemia (plasma cholesterol levels greater than 260 mg% [6.7 mmol/L]) were based on the 95th percentile levels of these plasma lipids in a normal population distribution from a Westernized culture.

These values have biostatistical relevance with respect to physiologic plasma cholesterol and triglyceride distributions around our population's mean levels. However, they fall short of a public health related measurement with therapeutic implications aimed at establishing an ideal plasma cholesterol value for the purpose of lowering CAD risk.

Armed with recent evidence supporting the cholesterol hypothesis, the National Cholesterol Education Program Expert Panel has established more aggressive guidelines for defining hypercholesterolemia. This panel suggests that a plasma cholesterol level exceeding 240 mg% (6.21 mmol/L) is high, with a desirable level being that below 200 mg% (5.17 mmol/L). Similar guidelines of the European Atherosclerosis Society are also presented in this text.

Because of the increasing plasma cholesterol mortality slope of the curve shown by the MRFIT findings (Figure 1.1) at plasma cholesterol values above 200 mg% (5.2 mmol/L), plasma cholesterol values falling in the 200 to 239 mg% range (5.17 to 6.18 mmol/L) should be considered as suboptimally high, particularly when occurring in the presence of either:

- Personal history of definite CAD
- Two or more CAD risk factors

The current definition of hypercholesterolemia represents a compromise between providing a distinct definition of hypercholesterolemia based on normal distribution curves and a more clinically relevant zone of significant hypercholesterolemic values based on CAD risk likelihood. Because the presence of multiple CAD risk factors affects CAD risk in a synergistic manner, plasma cholesterol values assume increased importance in the presence of additional CAD risk factors.

Although a cholesterol value below 200 mg% (5.2 mmol/L) probably represents a desirable value in Western cultures, an ideal plasma cholesterol level remains to be clearly established. However, data from international epidemiological studies suggests that this range may be 120 to 180 mg% (3.1 to 4.7 mmol/L).

Patient Management

In terms of patient management, it should be recognized that measurement of total cholesterol alone does not fully reflect CAD risk on an individual basis. Consideration of the atherogenic plasma LDL-C component provides a better indication. Therefore, the current guidelines, which establish plasma LDL-C levels of less than 130 mg% (3.4 mmol/L) as desirable, are clearly preferable to using total cholesterol alone to gauge both population and personal CAD risk.

Similarly, the use of the plasma HDL-C level and total-cholesterol/HDL-C ratios (which combine the CAD risk considerations of atherogenic and protective lipid values) is also important in determining an individual's CAD risk, especially at average levels of plasma cholesterol. HDL-C determinations appear to lose their relevance with respect to CAD risk at extreme (low or high) plasma LDL-C levels.

Certainly, the current guidelines are preferable to the prior hypercholesterolemic levels based purely on population distributions. Employing these more recently established guidelines provides a more clinically relevant basis for the management of lipid disorders directed at CAD risk reduction. These recommendations are discussed in more detail in Section #19.

FIGURE 3.1 – **Relationship of Total Serum Cholesterol to CAD Risk**

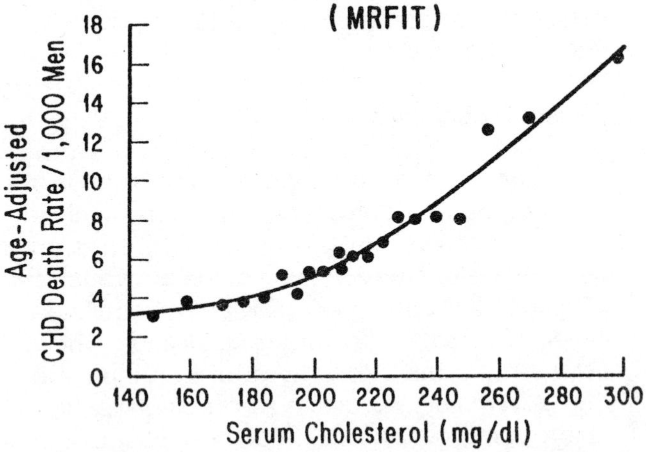

Serum cholesterol level and CAD mortality incidence in MRFIT subjects.

(Modified from Lancet 1986;2:933, reprinted with permission.)

References

The Expert Panel: Report of the National Cholesterol Education Program Expert Panel on Detection, Evaluation and Treatment of High Blood Cholesterol in Adults. Arch Intern Med 1988;148:36.

Frederickson DS, Levy RI, Lees RS: Fat transport in lipoproteins, an integrated approach to mechanisms and disorders. N Engl J Med 1967;276:148.

Grundy SM, Goodman DWS, et al: The place of HDL in cholesterol management: a perspective from the National Cholesterol Education Program. Arch Intern Med 1989;149:505.

Marmot MG: Hypercholesterolemia: a public health problem. Atheroscler Rev 1988;18:95.

Olson RE: A critique of the report of the National Institutes of Health Expert Panel of Detection, Evaluation and Treatment of High Blood Cholesterol. Arch Intern Med 1989;149:1501.

#4 Lipoprotein Metabolism

4.

Lipids and Lipoproteins

Cholesterol and triglycerides (fats) are the major body lipids, with important biological functions (Figure 4.1). Cholesterol is used for:

- Cell structure
- Precursor for synthesis of a variety of steroid hormones

Triglyceride fat serves in:

- Cell structure
- Provision of the body's major energy source

Lipids are nonpolar compounds and, therefore, not soluble in water. Because the blood is an aqueous medium, the formation of lipoprotein complexes is required in order to transport lipids to the tissue cells, where they can be utilized.

Lipoprotein particles are formed by combining cholesterol and triglycerides with phospholipids and apolipoproteins. Five major fractions of lipoprotein particles are identified according to their density, determined by ultracentrifugation (Figure 4.1).

Lipoprotein Classes

Chylomicrons
(Density Less Than 0.95)

Chylomicrons are derived from dietary (exogenous) fats, absorbed from the intestine, and formed in the intestinal epithelium. These particles consist largely of triglycerides (98 percent by weight) with cholesterol and a unique apolipoprotein B-48.

Chylomicrons are hydrolyzed at the capillary surface with the removal of triglycerides from the lipid core of the particle. The triglycerides are removed by tissue lipases, which require apolipoprotein C-II as a cofactor.

The triglycerides provide energy for skeletal muscles' use and for adipocyte storage. The remaining (or remnant) particle (relatively rich in cholesterol esters) is responsible for carrying dietary fats (100 g triglyceride and 500 mg cholesterol daily) to the liver where they can be utilized further as shown in Figure 4.2.

Chylomicron remnants are recognized and removed from the plasma by hepatic receptors containing apo-E. The rate of clearance of remnant particles depends upon which subfraction of apo-E is present. Particles containing apo-E_2 are removed more slowly than those with apo-E_3 and apo-E_4.

Very Low-Density Lipoprotein **(VLDL)**
(Density 0.95 to 1.006)

This particle, consisting largely of triglycerides, is secreted by the hepatocyte and contains apolipoprotein B-100. Elevated VLDL levels are reflected by hypertriglyceridemia.

Triglycerides are removed from the circulating plasma VLDL-C particle by tissue lipases (delipidation) for storage (adipose lipoprotein lipase) or utilization (skeletal lipoprotein lipase). Apolipoprotein C has an important role in modulating lipoprotein lipase activity.

Intermediate Density Lipoproteins (IDL)
(Density 1.006 to 1.019)

These particles, formed transiently during VLDL catabolism, are also referred to as beta-VLDL or VLDL remnants. They contain apo-E and are removed by the liver through the LDL (or B/E) receptor.

The condition of dysbetalipoproteinemia (Type III hyperlipoproteinemia) is a lipid disorder characterized by the abnormal presence of plasma IDL. This condition is due to a defective apolipoprotein E (apo-E_2 isoform) in conjunction with an over-production of VLDL, causing the accumulation of the uncatabolized remnant IDL which is characteristic of this disorder.

In this setting, there is an impedance in the usual pathways of IDL metabolism, involving direct hepatic uptake of IDL, or its conversion to LDL. The remnant particles appear to be atherogenic.

Low-Density Lipoprotein (LDL)
(Density 1.019 to 1.063)

This is a relatively cholesterol-enriched compound compared with its VLDL precursor. This particle is the major cholesterol-furnishing source and cholesterol-carrying lipoprotein and can be catabolized by both receptor- and nonreceptor-mediated pathways.

The presence of LDL receptors has been identified in coated pits on cell surfaces for the purpose of LDL uptake. This process is mediated via apolipoprotein B-100 and/or apo-E, allowing subsequent cellular cholesterol acquisition and utilization of cholesterol for cell needs (i.e., B/E receptors).

It is important to recognize that 70 percent of LDL-C receptors are found on the hepatocytes, allowing the liver to reutilize cholesterol. The cholesterol brought into cells by this receptor-mediated process curbs further cholesterol synthesis by inhibiting activity of the rate-limiting enzyme of cholesterol synthesis, 3-hydroxy-3-methylglutaryl-coenzyme A (HMG-CoA) reductase. This allows the cells a method of regulating their cholesterol content. For example, the dietary cholesterol from the chylomicron remnant particles is thought to down-regulate the hepatic LDL receptors.

The nonreceptor-mediated pathway of LDL-C utilization represents a scavenger route involving the macrophages of the reticuloendothelial system. This pathway, which appears to be particularly responsive to the accumulation of modified LDL-C, has been implicated in the atherogenic process.

Modified LDL-C represents both LDL-C particles that have been oxidized by free radicals or glycosylated. These important chemical alterations increase LDL-C atherogenicity. Probucol, probably acting as an antioxidant, slows progression of atherosclerotic lesions in the Watanabe rabbit model.

Familial Hypercholesterolemia has been identified as a Mendelian autosomal dominant disorder resulting from the presence of an LDL receptor defect. Elevated plasma LDL-C levels occur in this condition because cellular uptake of plasma LDL-C is reduced. Familial Hypercholesterolemia is characterized by extremely elevated total (LDL and IDL) plasma cholesterol levels that are atherogenic.

High-Density Lipoprotein (HDL)
(Density greater than or equal to 1.063)

This particle contains apolipoprotein A and participates in "reverse cholesterol" transport, as illustrated in Figure 4.3. HDL is formed from nascent HDL, which coalesce to form discoid particles rich in apolipoprotein corresponding with the HDL_3 subfraction (density 1.125 to 1.210). This particle is transformed into the less dense, spherical HDL_2 sub-fraction (density 1.063 to 1.125), which is filled with cholesterol esters.

This process of HDL maturation (HDL-cholesterol acquisition from peripheral tissues) involves the activation of lecithin cholesterol acyltransferase (LCAT) by apolipoprotein A-1. LCAT esterifies free cholesterol that has been removed from peripheral tissues by HDL_3, allowing transport of this esterified molecule in HDL_2, which in turn delivers cholesterol directly to the liver where it can be eliminated through the biliary system.

Besides this classic reverse transport pathway, HDL-C also transfers cholesterol to VLDL-C and LDL-C in exchange for triglycerides. This is a more recently established reverse transport process, which indirectly enables this HDL transferred cholesterol to be returned to the liver's hepatic LDL-C receptors via plasma LDL-C. Participation in the reverse transport process has been suggested as the mechanism by which HDL-C appears to be inversely associated with reduced CAD risk, although recent evidence suggests HDL has an antioxidant role which serves to prevent atherogenic LDL-oxidation. The HDL_2 subparticle has been generally regarded as the specific antiatherogenic component of HDL, this is not fully established; recent prospective evidence suggests the HDL_3 subparticle is as protective. Alternatively, HDL can be classified as those which contain only apo A-I (Lp A-I) and those which contain both apo A-I and apo A-II (LpA-I: A-II). Current evidence suggests LpA-I represents the beneficial HDL subparticle.

In addition, triglyceride metabolism is inversely linked with HDL metabolism. Hypertriglyceridemia causes plasma HDL-C_2 levels to be depressed. This may account for the effect of hypertriglyceridemia as a CAD risk factor.

Apolipoproteins

Table 4.1 summarizes the known functions of the major, currently-recognized apolipoproteins. The relationship of apolipoproteins to CAD risk is discussed in Section #28.

References

Brown MS, Goldstein JL: A receptor-mediated pathway for cholesterol homeostasis. Science 1986;232.

Cambien F, Parra HJ, Arvelier D, et al: Lipoprotein particles in patients with myocardial infarction and controls. Circulation 1990;82:III-348.

Havel RJ: Familial dysbetalipoproteinemia. Med Clin North Am 1982;66:441.

Jackson RL, Morrisett JD, Gotto AM: Lipoprotein structure and metabolism. Physiol Rev 1976;56: 259.

Kita T, Nagano Y, Yokode M, et al: Probucol prevents the progression of atherosclerosis in Watanabe heritable hyperlipemic rabbit. Proc Natl Acad Sci USA 1987;84:5928.

Parthasarathy S, Barnett J, Fong LG: High density lipoprotein inhibits the oxidative modification of low-density lipoprotein. Biochem Biophys Acta 1990;1044:275.

Purchois P, Kardoussi A, Fievet P, et al: Apolipoprotein A-I containing lipoprotein particles in coronary artery disease. Atherosclerosis 1987;68:35.

Reichi D, Miller NE: Pathophysiology of reverse cholesterol transport: insights from inherited disorders of lipid metabolism. Arteriosclerosis 1989; 9:785.

Rosenfeld ME: Oxidized LDL affects multiple atherogenic cellular responses. Circulation 1991;6:2137.

Smith DM: HDL system: a short review of structure and metabolism. Atheroscler Rev 1987;16:1.

Smith LC, Pownall HJ, Gotto AM: The plasma lipoproteins: structure and metabolism. Ann Rev Biochem 1978;47:751.

Stampfer MJ, Sacks FM, Salvinis CT, et al: A prospective study of cholesterol apolipoproteins and the risk of myocardial infarction. N Engl J Med 1991;325:373.

Steinberg D, Parthasarathy S, et al: Modifications of low-density lipoprotein that increase its atherogenicity. N Engl J Med 1989;320:915.

TABLE 4.1 – **Apolipoprotein Type**

Apolipoprotein Type	**Function**
A-I	Activates LCAT
B-48	Chylomicron formation
B-100	LDL-receptor recognition
C-II	Lipoprotein lipase activation
C-III	Lipoprotein lipase inhibition
E	Receptor activity for lipoprotein particle uptake
Transfer proteins	Facilitate the exchange of triglycerides, phospholipids and cholesterol esters between lipoprotein particles
Apo-(a)	Implicated in increased CAD risk

FIGURE 4.1 — **Structure of Cholesterol and Triglycerides**

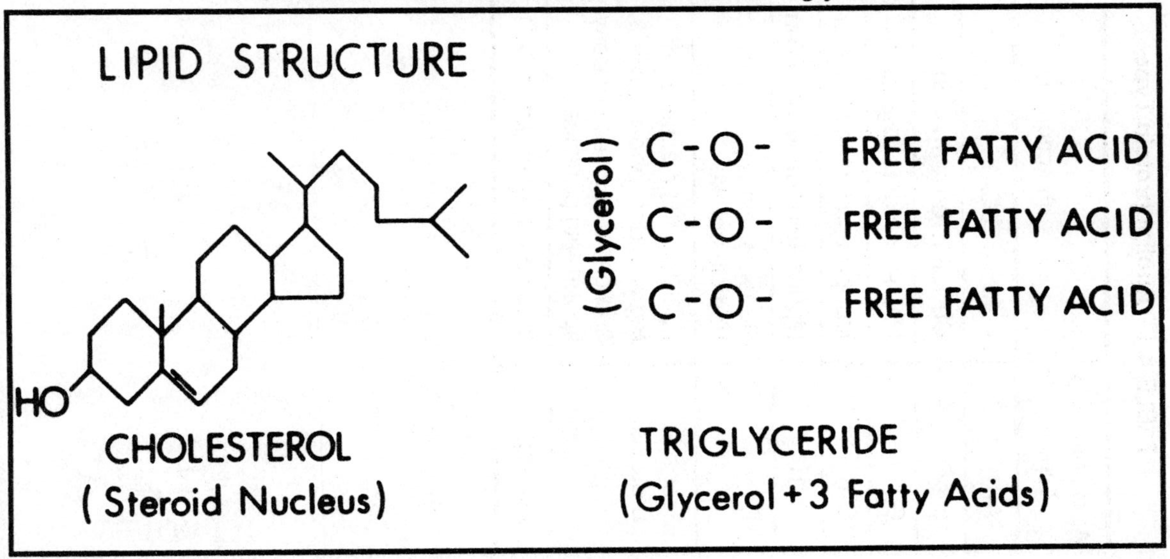

FIGURE 4.2—**LDL-C Metabolic Pathways**

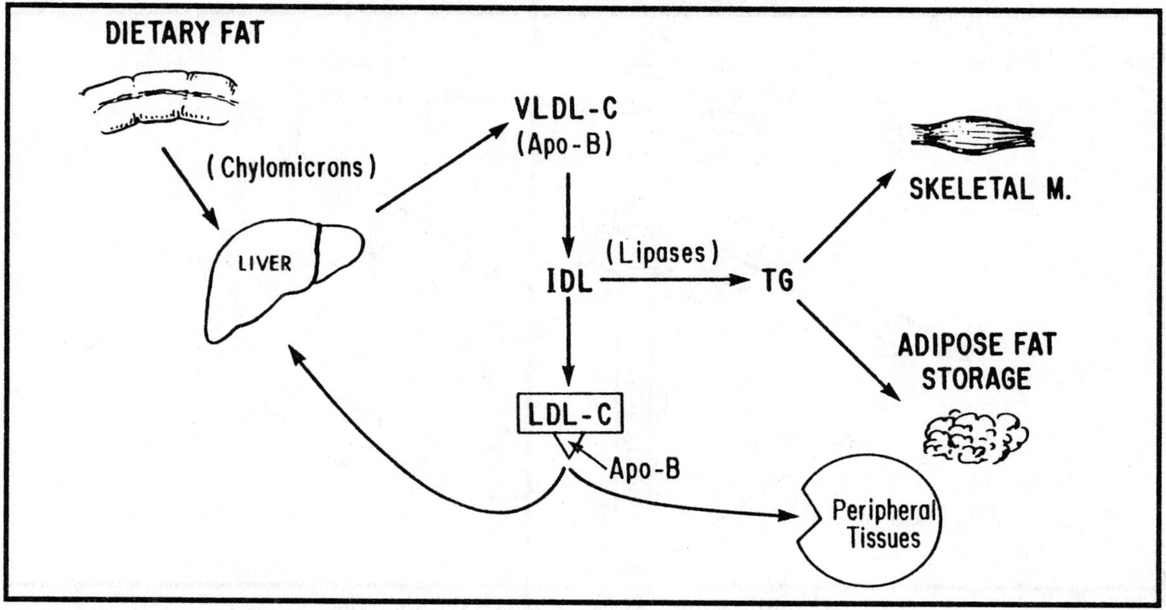

FIGURE 4.3 — **HDL-C Metabolic Pathways**

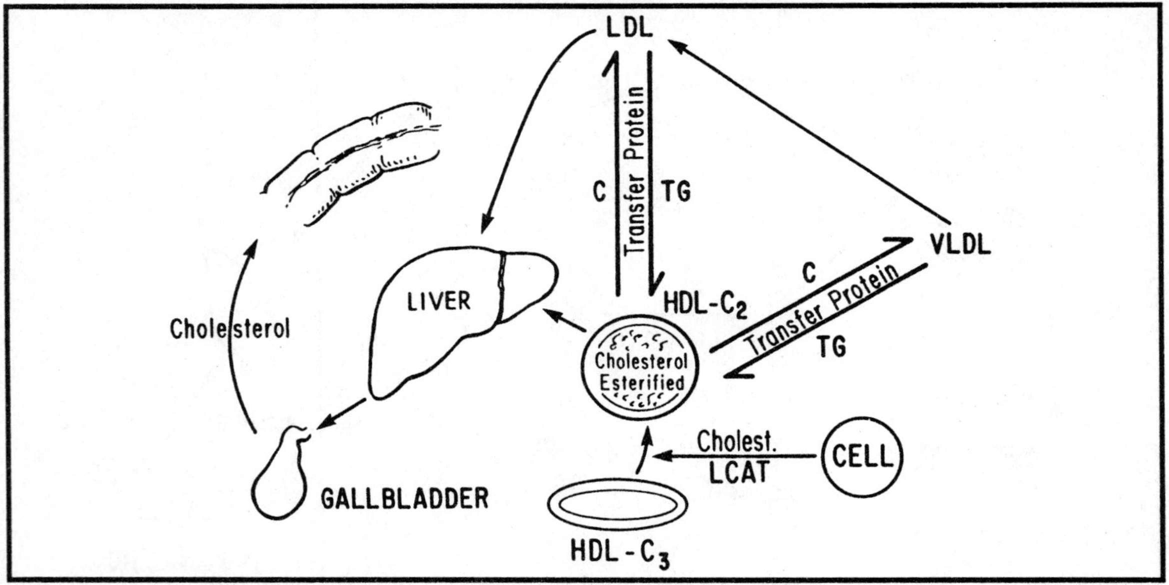

NOTES

#5 Classification of Lipid Disorders

Classification Systems

Various approaches have been used to describe lipid disorders, of which the simplest are primary (inherited) and secondary (acquired). The Frederickson-Levy classification, conversely, is the most well-established classification scheme, based purely on phenotypic (descriptive) characteristics of blood lipid levels. The European Atherosclerosis Society has also presented a recent clinicially formulated classification system also provided in this text.

5.

More recently, with improved understanding of lipid disorder metabolism, the classification of lipid disorders based on functional and genetically determined metabolic defects has been developed. As knowledge of the management of lipid disorders becomes more refined, especially with the advent of pharmaceutic compounds that have specific activities at particular points of the lipoprotein metabolic pathways, genotypically based classification schemes will continue to become more useful from the clinical standpoint.

Fredrickson-Levy Classification

The Fredrickson-Levy classification system for lipid disorders is shown in Table 5.1. The weakness of this system is that these disorders do not represent specific medical diagnoses. For example, a Type V patient who is treated for severe hypertriglyceridemia may be phenotypically converted to a Type IIb, III or IV patient once chylomicronemia is abolished.

Conversely, this patient becomes a Type V again if the condition is exacerbated. In addition, the Frederickson-Levy system does not account for plasma HDL-C levels, which are becoming more relevant to the practitioner as understanding of the relationship of plasma lipoproteins to CAD risk has grown.

Genotypic Classification

A more clinically useful scheme for the classification of lipid disorders based on the causation of the specific plasma lipid abnormality is described in more detail in Sections #6 and #7, but it is introduced here in order to compare it with the Frederickson-Levy system.

This system recognizes dyslipidemias to be of primary or secondary causes. Among the primary causes of lipid disorders, the common dyslipidemias are listed in Table 5.2 with their potential classification patterns according to the Frederickson system.

Given the recognition that lipid metabolic disorders can present such varied Frederickson-Levy types and the growing armamentarium of "designer" medications aimed at effecting specific steps of the metabolic pathways, the categorization schemes presented in the next two sections will continue to become more clinically relevant to the practitioner.

References

Frederickson DS, Levy RI, Lees RS: Fat transport in lipoproteins, an integrated approach to mechanisms and disorders. N Engl J Med 1967;276:148.

TABLE 5.1 — **Phenotypic (Fredrickson) Classification System With Characteristic Lipoprotein Abnormalities**

Classification	Lipoprotein Particle Abnormality
Type I	Chylomicron present
Type IIa	Elevated LDL — (cholesterol ≥ 250 mg%)
Type IIb	Elevated LDL — (cholesterol ≥ 250 mg%) Elevated VLDL — (triglycerides ≥ 250 mg%)
Type III	IDL present (broad band)
Type IV	Elevated VLDL — (triglycerides ≥ 250 mg%)
Type V	Elevated VLDL with the presence of chylomicronemia

TABLE 5.2 – **Major Genetic Dyslipidemias and Their Phenotypic Expressions**

Dyslipidemia	Potential Frederickson Presentation Type
Familial Hypercholesterolemia	IIa, IIb
Familial Hypertriglyceridemia	IV, V
Familial Combined Dyslipidemia	IIa, IIb, III, IV
Familial Dysbetalipoproteinemia	IIb, III, IV, V
Polygenic Hypercholesterolemia	IIa, IIb

TABLE 5.3—**Uncommon Dyslipidemias**

Disorder	Cause	Clinical
Abetalipoproteinemia	Congenital absence of apolipoprotein B (including both apo-B-100 and B-48 in the classic and homozygous forms)	Low plasma cholesterol and triglycerides, fat malabsorption with vitamin A, D, and E deficiency, ataxia, motor and sensory impairment, retinitis pigmentosa, acanthocytosis
Familial hypoalphalipoproteinemia	Autosomal dominant trait with HDL-C < 30 mg% in men and < 35 mg% in women	Increased CAD risk, not associated with corneal opacification. May be as frequent as one in 400 in the U.S. population
Tangier disease	Inherited absence or deficiency of HDL-C	Tissue accumulation of cholesterol esters. Orange, enlarged tonsils, splenomegaly, hepatomegaly, lymphadenopathy, neuromuscular dysfunction
Familial hyperalphalipoproteinemia	Primary HDL-C increase (> 70 mg% males, > 75 mg% females)	Reduced CAD risk, associated with the longevity syndrome

Familial LCAT deficiency	Increased free cholesterol levels in plasma	Corneal opacities, premature CAD, renal dysfunction
Familial apolipoprotein A-I and C-III deficiency	Inherited defect in apo-A-I and C-III synthesis	Corneal opacification with reduced plasma HDL-C levels. Prominent plantar xanthomas, premature CAD
Fish eye disease	Inherited metabolic defect resulting in apo-A-I and A-II reductions	Severe corneal opacification, reduced plasma HDL-C levels
Apo-A-I Milano	Cysteine for arginine base substitution on apo-A-I causing increased catabolism	Reduced plasma HDL-C level but without apparent increased CAD risk
Sitosterolemia	Autosomal recessive trait causing marked elevation of plant steroid levels	Development of tendon and tuberous xanthomas and premature CAD

6.

#6 Primary Dyslipidemias

Common Dyslipidemias

The following group of primary lipid disorders represents not only those disorders which are most frequently seen, but also most readily diagnosed by the practitioner. These dyslipidemias are listed in Table 5.2.

In contrast, the conditions presented in the second part of this discussion, which require highly specialized laboratory analytical methods to establish the diagnosis, are of less relevance to the practitioner.

Furthermore, the first group of lipid disorders presented is particularly important because they represent a group of conditions for which there exists available intervention therapy to treat the lipid disorder and potentially alter CAD mortality and morbidity risk. These disorders were introduced in the previous section and are presented here in more detail.

Familial Hypercholesterolemia

This is an autosomal dominant condition occurring in a heterozygotic (one in 500 occurrence) or homozygotic (one in a million occurrence) and resulting from the lack of monogenically controlled LDL-C receptor function. This includes individuals who are both receptor-negative and receptor-defective.

The homozygotic form is more severe, with physical evidence of elevated LDL-C levels present at birth (diagnosable by amniocentesis). This is reflected by the diffuse deposition of cholesteryl ester:

- Planar xanthomas
- Tendon xanthomas
- Corneal arcus with accelerated atherosclerosis – Leads to childhood CAD-related death

Plasma cholesterol values exceeding 700 mg% (18.1 mmol/L) are pathognomonic.

In the heterozygotic form, these clinical manifestations are delayed until early adulthood. Elevations of LDL-C are less pronounced than those noted in the homozygotic form and usually range between 300 and 500 mg% (7.6 to 12.9 mmol/L).

Clinically significant CAD events typically begin in men by the age of 50 years and somewhat later in women. The diagnosis can be confirmed by establishing severe hypercholesterolemia in family members according to the autosomal dominant mode of transmission. Tendon xanthomas, if present, are pathognomonic.

Familial Defective Apolipoprotein B-100

Familial defective apolipoprotein B-100 (FDB) is a recently recognized, dominantly inherited genetic disorder resulting from a mutation on the apo-B gene which produces a base substitution on the apo-B structure. This causes a reduced LDL affinity for the LDL receptor, resulting in an elevated plasma LDL-C to levels comparable with familial hypercholesterolemia. This is a serious disorder that leads to premature CAD. FDB can be diagnosed by molecular screening techniques and has an estimated occurrence of one in 600.

Familial Hypertriglyceridemias

This spectrum of diseases includes the extremely rare, recessive disorder involving lipoprotein lipase deficiency (Type I per the Frederickson classification) and resulting in severe hypertriglyceridemia in early childhood (the first week of life); it is dealt with in Section #25.

In contrast, the adult form of familial hypertriglyceridemia represents the outcome of either:

- Excessive hepatic VLDL production (triglycerides)
- Ineffective VLDL removal
- Both

This autosomal dominant disorder (one in 500 occurrence) occurs less frequently than secondary causes of hypertriglyceridemia and with elevated plasma VLDL (Type IV) or elevated plasma VLDL with chylomicronemia (Type V).

Characteristic clinical findings in the setting of chylomicronemia include:

- Eruptive xanthomas on:
  - Extensor surfaces
  - Abdomen
  - Buttocks
- Hepatomegaly
- Splenomegaly
- Lipemia retinalis

In addition, individuals suffering the following ailments are very sensitive to increases in body fat and dietary intake of fat, alcohol and estrogens, which may exacerbate:

- Acute pancreatitis (life-threatening concern)
- Abdominal discomfort (likely caused by distension of the viscera by triglyceride infiltration)

Familial Hyperchylomicronemia

Technically, this disorder should be classified as a hypertriglyceridemia, which presents with pure chylomicronemia lacking a concomitant elevation in plasma VLDL (Type I Frederickson). This disorder presents itself during infancy and childhood (see Section #25).

Familial Combined Hyperlipidemia

Resulting from hepatic overproduction of apolipoprotein B, this disorder by definition occurs with a variety of phenotypes in the first degree relatives: IIa, IIb, III and IV. This diagnosis is established by identifying the presence of differing phenotypically expressed lipid patterns in family members.

This is probably an autosomal dominant disorder and represents an increased CAD risk. Up to 20 percent of patients seen with this disorder experience a myocardial infarction before age 55.

Familial Dysbetalipoproteinemia (Broad Beta Disease)

Generally seen as a Type III, less often as a Type IV and rarely as a Type V phenotype, this condition represents the wide band of lipoprotein particles noted on plasma electrophoretic migration patterns termed "broad beta disease."

Typical plasma cholesterol values of 300 to 500 mg% (7.6 to 12.9 mmol/L) and triglyceride values of 400 to 700 mg% (4.5 to 7.9 mmol/L) are consistent with the IIb pattern. This finding reflects the presence of IDL in the plasma, resulting from an abnormality in apolipoprotein E in conjunction with an overproduction of VLDL (see Section #28).

The abnormal apolipoprotein alleles that result in the abnormal accumulation of plasma IDL particles are believed to bind dysfunctionally to LDL receptors. This impairs IDL and LDL catabolism and results in IDL accumulation.

The three known common alleles of apo-E are E_2, E_3 and E_4. These have been shown to differ by a single amino acid residue. This allows them to be separated by isoelectric focusing studies. Although the prevalence of culpable apo-E isoforms (E_2E_2) is not uncommon, the clinical manifestations of this disorder are seen in only approximately one in 10,000 individuals, thus implying the existence of a secondary defect (i.e., VLDL overproduction).

Yellow or orange palmar xanthomas are unique to this condition and are seen in nearly half of the patients.

Often occurring with this dyslipidemia are:

- Obesity
- Diabetes
- Manifestations of CAD

Increased risk for peripheral vascular disease in smokers is virtually a certainty. The diagnosis is established by serum electrophoresis to reveal the broad band or by beta quantification ultracentrifugation of the plasma to measure directly a

VLDL cholesterol/triglyceride ratio greater than three to 10 (i.e., VLDL-C/triglyceride ratio exceeding 0.3) (see Section #2).

Familial Polygenic Hypercholesterolemia

Although this condition has an acknowledged inheritance component, the term "polygenic" is employed in order to indicate that this disorder does not represent the outcome of a single gene defect. This concomitantly masks ignorance as to the etiology of the most common lipid disorder seen by the practitioner which likely represents a group of several distinct patterns of LDL metabolism. This polygenic form of hypercholesterolemia is the most common dyslipidemia and occurs frequently.

Analogous to essential hypertension, this condition accounts for well over 95 percent of hypercholesterolemics. Usually plasma cholesterol elevations noted in these patients are below those seen in familial hypercholesterolemia (typical range 200 to 350 mg% [5.2 to 9.1 mmol/L]).

Phenotypically, as either Type IIa or IIb, a large percentage of these individuals are readily therapeutically responsive to dietary fat restriction appropriately referred to as hyper-responders.

Although the diagnosis may seem banal, this condition represents the most important lipid disorder from the public health standpoint, justifying national approaches to effecting large-scale reductions in the current approximate plasma cholesterol mean of 210 mg% (5.4 mmol/L) to a goal of at least below 200 mg% (5.2 mmol/L). This requires effort of both widespread public education and individualized medical care.

Uncommon Dyslipidemias

Table 5.3 summarizes other currently recognized conditions resulting from unusual disorders in lipid metabolism.

References

Brunzell JD, Albers JJ, et al: Plasma lipoproteins in familial combined hyperlipidemia and monogenic familial hypertriglyceridemia. J Lipid Res 1983;24:147.

Frederickson DS, Morganroth J, Levy RI: Type III hyperlipoproteinemia: an analysis of two contemporary definitions. Ann Intern Med 1975;82:150.

Goldstein JL, Schrott HG, et al: Hyperlipidemia in coronary heart disease. J Clin Invest 1973;52:1544.

Gregg RE, Zech LA, et al: Type III hyperlipoproteinemia: defective metabolism of an abnormal apolipoprotein E. Science 1981;211:584.

Grundy SM, Chait A, Brunzell JD: Familial combined hyperlipidemia workshop. Arteriosclerosis 1987;7:203.

Hazzard WR, Warnick R, et al: Genetic transmission of isoapolipoprotein E phenotypes in a large kindred. Metabolism 1981;30:79.

Illingworth DR, Connor WE: Disorders in lipid metabolism. In: Endocrinology and Metabolism, 2nd ed. Felig P, Baxter JD, Broadus AE, Frohman LA (eds.) New York: McGraw-Hill, 1987.

Mabuchi H, Koizumi J, et al: Development of coronary heart disease in familial hypercholesterolemia. Circulation 1989;79:225.

Morganroth J, Levy RI, Frederickson DS: The biochemical, clinical and genetic features of Type III hyperlipoproteinemia. Ann Intern Med 1975;82:158.

Motulsky AG: Current concepts in genetics: the genetic hyperlipidemias. N Engl J Med 1976;294:83.

Sane T, Nikkilä EA: Very low density lipoprotein triglyceride metabolism in relatives of hypertriglyceridemic probands. Arteriosclerosis 1988;8: 217.

Tybjaerg-Hansen A, Gallagher J, et al: Familial defective apolipoprotein B-100: detection in the United Kingdom and Scandinavia, and clinical characteristics of ten cases. Arteriosclerosis 1990;80:235.

Vega GL, Denke MA, Grundy SM: Metabolic basis of primary hypercholesterolemia. Circulation 1991;84:118.

Williams KJ, Petrie KA, Brocia RW, Swenson TL: Lipoprotein lipase modulates net secretory output of apolipoprotein B in vitro. A possible pathophysiologic explanation of familial combined hyperlipidemia. J Clin Invest 1991;88:1300.

#7 Secondary Causes of Dyslipidemia

Medical Causes

Dyslipidemic conditions can frequently result from associated medical conditions. Because secondary dyslipidemia can often be corrected by treatment of the underlying disease, the presence of dyslipidemia justifies testing to rule out the more common diseases. Examples of these possible causes and their corresponding screening procedures are as follows:

7.

- Diabetes mellitus – Fasting blood glucose
- Obstructive liver disease – Alkaline phosphatase
- Hypothyroidism – Serum TSH
- Nephrotic Syndrome – Urinalysis (albumin)

Potential medical causes of dyslipidemia less common than those previously mentioned include:

- Acute intermittent porphyria
- Anorexia nervosa
- AIDS
- Cholestasis
- Cushing's syndrome
- Dysglobulinemias
- Glycogenesis
- Hepatic failure
- Hypopituitarism
- Lipodystrophies
- Organ transplant
- Renal diseases and dialysis
- Stress
- Systemic lupus erythematosus
- Uremia

Lipid Levels Affected by Medication

A number of commonly used medications can influence plasma lipid levels. Although technically not a medication, ethanol consumption represents a common cause of hypertriglyceridemia.

Glucocorticoid and estrogen-containing medications tend to raise plasma triglyceride levels. Estrogens have a beneficial increasing effect on HDL-C, whereas progestinal agents tend to lower plasma HDL-C levels. The effects of Tamoxifen mirror those of estrogens except they have a less pronounced HDL-C raising effect. Also 13-*cis*-retinoic acid (Accutane®), (used in skin preparations) can raise triglycerides. Anabolic steroid use also lowers plasma HDL-C levels.

Commonly used anti-hypertensive agents can paradoxically have adverse effects on the lipoprotein profile. The use of these agents in major clinical trials involving treatment of hypertension has been suggested as a potential reason for the lack of anticipated CAD risk-reducing outcome of these trials because of concomitant adverse effects on plasma lipids and lipoproteins.

Hydrochlorothiazide and loop diuretics tend to raise plasma triglyceride and LDL-C levels. Non-selective beta blockers lower HDL-C (HDL_2 subfraction) levels. Because hypertension frequently coexists with hypercholesterolemia, the clinician should select a class of anti-hypertensive agents which is lipid neutral such as:

- Selective beta blocker
- Alpha-1 antagonist
- ACE inhibitor
- Calcium channel blocker

References

Avram MM, et al: Cholesterol and lipid disturbances in renal disease: the natural history of uremic dyslipidemia and the impact of hemodialysis and continous ambulatory peritoneal dialysis. Am J Med 1989;87:5.

Glazer G: Atherogenic effects of anabolic steroids on serum lipid levels. A literature review. Arch Intern Med 1991;151:1925.

Grundy SM, Vega GL: Rationale and management of hyperlipidemia in the nephrotic syndrome. Am J Med 1989;87:5.

Grunfeld C, Kotler DP, Shigenaga JK, et al: Circulating Interferon-alpha levels and hypertriglyceridemia in acquired immunodeficiency syndrome. Am J Med 1991;90:154.

Havel RJ: Approach to the patient with hyperlipidemia. Med Clin N Amer 1982;66:319.

Lardinois CK, Neuman SL: The effect of antihypertensive agents on lipids and lipoproteins. Arch Intern Med 1988;148:1280.

Love RR, Wiebe DA, Newcomb PA, et al: Effects of tamoxifen on cardiovascular risk factors in women. Ann Intern Med 1991;115:860.

Markell MS, Friedman EA: Hyperlipidemia after organ transplantation. Am J Med;1989:87:5.

Weinberger MH: Anti-hypertensive therapy and lipids: paradoxical influences on cardiovascular disease risk. Am J Med 1986;80(2A):60.

#8 Decision For Use of Cholesterol-Lowering Agents

When to Use Medications

The decision to use cholesterol-lowering agents is based on the lack of success in achieving adequate plasma LDL-C levels after six months of dietary intervention (see Section #19). The six month period may be shortened in high-risk circumstances, e.g., evidence of advanced CAD or the presence of familial hypercholesterolemia.

Medication is then required for plasma LDL-C greater than:

- 160 mg% (4.1 mmol/L) in high-risk patients
- 190 mg% (4.9 mmol/L) in non-high-risk patients

8.

Based on current evidence from regression studies, a more aggressive approach ultimately aimed at reducing LDL-C below 100 mg% (2.6 mmol/L) is warranted in patients with documented CAD.

Selection of Medication

Medications should be selected on the basis of the lipid disorder to be managed (see Sections #10 through #14). Medication doses should be gradually advanced with cautious attention to the appearance of possible side effects.

Plasma LDL-C levels should be used to monitor therapy for hypercholesterolemia and checked at six-week intervals until a stable, therapeutic LDL-C goal level is achieved.

NOTES

#9 Hypertriglyceridemia

Definition

According to the Frederickson classification based on the 95th percentile as the cutoff, hypertriglyceridemia occurs when plasma triglyceride levels exceed 250 mg% (2.8 mmol/L). Specific guidelines to define hypertriglyceridemia with respect to CAD risk remain to be firmly established. However, the European Guidelines which base CAD risk on non-HDL-C plasma cholesterol levels (ie, VLDL-C + LDL-C) indirectly incorporate plasma triglycerides into the CAD risk equation. Severe hypertriglyceridemia with the presence of fasting chylomicronemia has recognized medical importance for its relationship to acute pancreatitis.

Hypertriglyceridemia and CAD risk

The relationship of plasma triglyceride levels to CAD risk is highly controversial. Although early studies evidenced a direct relationship of increasing plasma triglyceride levels to CAD risk, this association has not been borne out by more sophisticated analytical methods involving multivariate regression techniques. In addition, a prospective triglyceride lowering intervention trial remains to be initiated.

Plasma triglyceride levels are typically associated with other potential confounding variables for CAD risk, including:

- Low plasma HDL-C levels
- Diabetes mellitus
- Obesity

When these variables are entered into multivariate regression equations, plasma triglyceride levels have not been unequivocally shown to be an independent CAD risk factor in men. However, recent findings from the Framingham Heart Study indicate that hypertriglyceridemia is an independent CAD risk factor for women.

Perhaps a more appropriate manner of viewing this relationship is to recognize that hypertriglyceridemia does not represent a single disease entity. Clearly, Type III dyslipidemia is associated with increased CAD risk, as are familial combined dyslipidemias with IIb, III or IV patterns, i.e., reflecting the presence of hypertriglyceridemia.

Thus, the heterogeneity of these hypertriglyceridemic lipid disorders is another reason for its lack of statistical correlation with large-scale CAD risk factor studies. Current evidence suggests that the VLDL and chylomicron remnant particles represent the atherogenic "triglyceride particles." Further research is needed to clarify these relationships and related pathogenic mechanisms.

Hypertriglyceridemia Therapeutic Goals – Acute Pancreatitis

In cases of severe hypertriglyceridemia with the presence of fasting chylomicronemia usually occurring with plasma triglyceride levels in excess of 1,000 mg% (11.3 mmol/L) (Type V), immediate intervention is required to abolish chylomicronemia and eliminate any immediate risk from acute pancreatitis. This medical emergency is best treated by a no-fat hypocaloric diet (rice, fruit, etc.) and may require hospitalization to ensure compliance and monitor outcome. When the patient is experiencing symptoms of acute pancreatitis, they should be placed NPO, receiving only intravenous dextrose and saline solution until the chylomicronemia clears.

Insulin administration is also useful in lower ing plasma triglyceride levels in diabetic patients in a medically controlled setting. Once chylomicronemia has cleared, long-term dietary goals should include:

- Reduced fat intake
- Restriction of ethanol-containing beverages (which raise plasma triglyceride levels)
- Weight loss in conjunction with a regular exercise program
- Avoiding estrogen medications

This requires long-term monitoring. During pregnancy these patients should be closely monitored on a strict low-fat diet. Because these individuals are highly sensitive to dietary fat intake, long-term medication use is appropriate to maintain triglyceride values at least below 500 mg% (5.6 mmol/L), with an ideal value below 150 mg% (1.7 mmol/L). This is because a hypertriglyceridemic patient can experience greater postprandial triglyceride swings to levels well above those reflected by fasting lipoprotein values.

CAD

The recommendations for triglyceride-lowering therapy at lower plasma triglyceride levels are not well established. Appropriate lipid disorders requiring aggressive plasma triglyceride management are those of Types IIb, III and IV, especially when there is an underlying personal or family history of CAD or diabetes mellitus.

Because plasma triglyceride reduction causes reciprocal plasma HDL-C increases, this is an especially worthwhile intervention when plasma HDL-C levels are depressed. Because of recent Framingham Study evidence, hypertriglyceridemia in women should be definitively acted upon, especially in the presence of diabetes mellitus.

Therapy includes a diet restricted in fat intake (Step 2) with weight loss when needed. Physical activity pursuits are an important means for reducing triglycerides and raising plasma HDL-C levels. Improved insulin control is also important for the diabetic. Although specific guidelines are not firmly established, a therapeutic goal of 150 mg% (1.7 mmol/L) should be the targeted triglyceride level. A minimum goal should be to keep plasma triglycerides below 250 mg% (2.8 mmol/L), especially for the patient who is at high CAD risk.

References

Austin MA: Plasma triglyceride and coronary heart disease. Arterio and Throm 1991;11:2.

Brunzell JD, Bierman EL: Chylomicronemia syndrome. Med Clin North Am 1982;66:468.

Connor WE, Connor SL: The dietary treatment of hyperlipidemia. Med Clin North Am 1982;66:485.

Hulley JB, Rosenman RH, et al: The association between triglycerides and coronary heart disease. N Engl J Med 1980;302:1383.

Kannel WB: Metabolic risk factors for coronary heart disease in women: A perspective from the Framingham Study. Am Heart J 1987;114:413.

Leaf DA: Hypertriglyceridemia: Assessment and management of the other lipid disorders. Medical Rounds 1988;1:259.

Santamarina-Fojo S, Brewer HB: The Familial Hyperchylomicronemic syndrome. New insights into underlying genetic defects. JAMA 1991;265:904.

NOTES

#10 Bile Acid Sequestrants

Clinical Information

This category of plasma LDL-C-reducing agents includes cholestyramine (Questran®) and colestipol (Colestid®). These remain the first choice of medication for isolated hypercholesterolemia (Type IIa), particularly the polygenic forms. An exception for use of these medications would be for patients with severe constipation.

Because they are not absorbed into the system, bile acid sequestrants are currently the only medications considered safe for children. The use of cholestyramine has been shown to be effective in lowering cholesterol levels and CAD risk by the Lipid Research Clinic trial.

Mode of Action

Bile acid sequestrants bind bile acids in the intestine and interrupt the enterohepatic circulation of bile acids. This increases cholesterol excretion from the gastrointestinal tract. The depletion of hepatic cholesterol serves to stimulate increased hepatic LDL-C receptor activity, ultimately causing reduction in plasma LDL-C levels.

This medication is less effective in patients with homozygotic familial hypercholesterolemia because they completely lack underlying LDL-C receptor activity. This is not true for the more common heterozygotic forms, which retain partial receptor function.

A potential concern in patients with concurrent hypertriglyceridemia (IIb) is the compensatory hepatic increase in plasma VLDL-C levels, which accompanies the administration of bile acid sequestrants. This can result in concomitant elevations of plasma triglyceride levels in association with LDL-C reduction, which can potentially provoke an episode of acute pancreatitis.

Clinical Use

These medications should be initiated in fractional dosages and gradually advanced as needed to a maximum quantity of 15 g colestipol BID, or 12 g cholestyramine BID (5 g colestipol = 4 g cholestyramine). These medications are available as powders and should be taken as a slurry mixed with water or juice.

Questran® Light, made with NutraSweet®, is a newly marketed low-calorie form of its parent. Cholybar® is a more recently available confectionery form which resembles a candy bar and may prove to be a more conveniently administered form of the medication.

Because they interfere with the absorption of anionic medications, these other medications should be taken one hour before or four hours following administration of the sequestrant. The sequestrant should be taken with or just after meals for optimal effect.

A non-linear dose response in plasma LDL-C reduction is observed in both medications, with a reduction of up to 20 percent in plasma LDL-C levels occurring with maximum dosages. Little additional benefit is gained from greater amounts, which are associated with increased incidence of gastrointestinal side effects. The use of these medications is restricted to patients with elevated LDL-C levels.

The concomitant use of niacin is helpful to blunt increased plasma VLDL-C levels in patients with the IIb phenotype who are treated with plasma LDL-C lowering agents. Thus, although bile acid sequestrants are most effective in the poly-genic form of hypercholesterolemia, they are less effective in patients with familial combined dyslipidemia (those who overproduce apolipoprotein B and VLDL-C) and not effective in patients with homozygotic forms of familial hypercholesterolemia who do not experience any LDL receptor up-regulation because they intrinsically lack receptor function. The medication has a significant but slight plasma HDL-C-increasing effect.

Side Effects

Possible side effects from use of bile acid sequestrants may include:

- Unpleasant texture inciting palatability-related complaints
- Changes in bowel function, such as:
  - Constipation
  - Nausea
  - Flatulence
  - Epigastric fullness
- Precipitation of intestinal obstruction (rare)
- Decreased absorption of fat-soluble vitamins A and D and folic acid (should be supplemented in children)
- Hyperchloremic acidosis, a rare metabolic complication
- Possibility of mild hypertriglyceridemia
- Mild abnormalities of liver function
- Loss of dental enamel

Decreases in drug availability may cause difficulties with administration of medication, the most commonly used being:

- Digoxin (Tubex®, Lanoxicaps®, Lanoxin®)
- Thyroxine (Euthroid®, Levothroid®, Synthroid®)
- Coumarin (Coumadin®, Panwarfin®)
- Thiazide diuretics

References

Brown MS, Goldstein JL: Drugs used in the treatment of hypercholesterolemias. In: The Pharmacological Basis of Therapeutics, 7th Ed. Gilman, et al (eds.) New York: Macmillan Publishing Co., 1985;827.

Curtis DM, Driscoll DJ, Goldman DH: Loss of dental enamel in a patient taking cholestyramine. Mayo Clin Proc 1991;66:1131.

Lipid Research Clinics Program: The Lipid Research Clinics Coronary Primary Prevention Trial Results I. Reduction in incidence of coronary heart disease; and II. The relationship of reduction in incidence of coronary heart disease to cholesterol lowering. JAMA 1986;251:351.

Schaefer EJ, Levy RI: Pathogenesis and management of lipoprotein disorders. N Engl J Med 1985;312:1300.

Shepherd J, Packard CJ, et al: Cholestyramine promotes receptor mediated low density lipoprotein catabolism. N. Engl J Med 1980;302:1219.

#11 Niacin

Clinical Introduction

Niacin is a medication with longstanding, documented, hypolipemic effects for both plasma triglycerides and cholesterol. With the development of more potent plasma LDL-C-active agents, the use of niacin for this purpose has decreased. Similarly, although effective in plasma triglyceride lowering, its use in these forms of dyslipidemia is becoming supplanted by gemfibrozil, which has fewer side effects.

Although compliance has been a longstanding issue with niacin use due to flushing and gastrointestinal side effects, long-term studies indicate that niacin use is associated with both reduced CAD events and overall mortality. Unfortunately, the reduced incidence of flushing evidenced by the newer sustained-release forms is offset by more severe gastrointestinal side effects (particularly hepatitis) which limits their total daily dosing level.

This form is less effective in lowering plasma triglycerides and raising HDL-C than the regular form. Although the use of niacin requires more physician skill and patient motivation than other medications and will probably be supplanted by other medications, it is important to recognize that this form of therapy is the least expensive and remains an important adjunctive medication for concomitant therapy with other primarily LDL-C-lowering agents.

Mode of Action

The mechanism(s) of action for niacin remains to be clearly defined, despite extensive research efforts. Niacin is acknowledged to reduce hepatocyte VLDL synthesis, which in turn reduces LDL-C production. Reduction of VLDL-C synthesis represents the outcome of decreased-lipolysis (and hence availability) of plasma-free fatty acids for:

- VLDL-C synthesis
- Hepatic esterification of triglyceride formation
- Reduced hepatic apolipoprotein-B production

The reduction of plasma VLDL-C levels is associated with concomitant increases in plasma HDL-C levels.

Clinical Use

Niacin is dispensed in 100 and 500 mg capsules with therapeutic effects achieved with 500 mg to 3 g TID, although a typically effective daily dose is 2 g. The primary side effects of this medication are:

- Prostaglandin-mediated cutaneous flushing
- Nausea
- Abdominal discomfort
- Diarrhea

These symptoms are best avoided by gradually increasing the therapeutic doses. However, patients receiving sustained-release forms of the medication are usually unable to tolerate more than two grams per day due to gastrointestinal side effects.

Begin with 100 mg TID after meals, with an increase of 100 mg with each dose each week for five weeks or until therapeutic levels are achieved.

The duration and magnitude of these complaints usually diminish with long-term therapy. The prostaglandin-mediated flushing effects can be blocked by the administration of an aspirin given 30 minutes prior to the medicative dose. The medication is tolerated better when taken with meals.

Because of the potential risk of niacin-induced hepatitis and increasing uric acid and glucose levels, liver function tests and uric acid and glucose levels should be checked as a premedication baseline and monitored frequently until a stable medication dose is achieved, and then periodically thereafter. A threefold increase of liver function tests above the laboratory upper limit of normal requires immediate cessation of the medication, although it may be cautiously reinstituted at a later time when this has resolved.

Niacin is contraindicated in patients with any one of the following:

- Active liver disease
- History of peptic ulcer disease
- Hyperuricemia

The medication should be used cautiously in diabetics, as it can aggravate glycemic control.

Macular edema, presenting as blurred vision, is reversible with discontinuation of the medication, as is acanthosis nigricans.

Anticipated changes in plasma lipids and lipoproteins with therapy include:

- Plasma LDL-C reduction – 15 to 25 percent
- Triglyceride reduction – 25 to 40 percent
- Plasma HDL-C increase – 30 to 35 percent

Side Effects

Use of niacin may result in any of the following possible side effects:

- Cutaneous flushing occurring between 15 minutes and two hours of administration, diminishing with prolonged therapy
- Gastrointestinal symptoms such as:
  - Nausea
  - Abdominal discomfort
  - Diarrhea
  - Activation of peptic ulcer disease
  - Liver function test abnormalities
  - Risk of hepatitis
- Enhancement in effects of vasodilatory and ganglioplegic antihypertensive agents, exacerbating vasodilatory and postural hypotensive effects
- Exacerbation of hyperuricemia
- Exacerbation of gout
- Macular edema with blurred vision
- Itching, rash, hyperpigmentation of the skin developing into acanthosis nigricans
- Aggravation of hyperglycemia in diabetes mellitus

The use of niacin through self prescription is irresponsible and should be discouraged.

References

Alderman JD, Pasternak RC: Effect of a modified, well-tolerated niacin regimen on serum total cholesterol, high density lipoprotein cholesterol and the cholesterol to high density lipoprotein ratio. Am J Cardiol 1989;64:725.

Brown WV, Goldberg IJ, Ginsberg HN: Treatment of common lipoprotein disorders. Prog Cardiovasc Dis 1984;27:1.

Canner PL, et al: Fifteen-year mortality in Coronary Drug Project patients: Long-term benefit with niacin. J Am Coll Cardiol 1986;8:1245.

Carlson LA, Rosenhamer G: Reduction of mortality in the Stockholm Ischaemic Heart Disease Secondary Prevention Study by combined treatment with clofibrate and nicotinic acid. Acta Med Scand 1988;223:405.

Etchason JA, Miller TD, Squires RW, et al: Niacin-induced hepatitis: A potential side effect with low-dose time-release niacin. Mayo Clin Proc 1991;66:23.

Grundy JM, Mok HYI, et al: The influence of nicotinic acid on metabolism of cholesterol and triglycerides in man. J Lipid Research 1981;22:24.

Henkin Y, Johnson KC, Segrest JP: Rechallenge with crystalline niacin after drug-induced hepatitis from sustained-release niacin. JAMA 1990;264:241.

Henkin Y, Obermon A, Hurst DC, et al: Niacin revisited: Clinical observations on an important but under-utilized drug. Am J Med 1991;91:239.

Knopp RH, et al: Contrasting effects of unmodified and time-release forms of niacin on lipoproteins in hyperlipidemic subjects: Clues to mechanism of action of niacin. Metabolism 1985;34:642.

#12 Fibric Acid Derivatives

Clinical Information

Although a number of fibric acid derivatives are under development, only two are currently approved for clinical use in the U.S.:

- Gemfibrozil (Lopid®)
- Clofibrate (Atromid-S®)

This discussion considers gemfibrozil because it has a track record clinically proven to be safer than clofibrate, which currently should be restricted to use as an agent of second choice.

The Helsinki Heart Study results have provided important evidence to expand the indications of gemfibrozil as the first drug of choice for all hypertriglyceridemic disorders except Type I (i.e., IIb, III, IV, V). This medication, which is typically given in a 600 mg BID dose, will probably supplant niacin in the general treatment of hypertriglyceridemia because it is well tolerated and has a consistent HDL-C-raising effect.

Mode of Action

The triglyceride-lowering effects of gemfibrozil are primarily caused by a reduction of hepatic synthesis of VLDL-C and apolipoprotein B, with a concomitant increase in the removal of triglyceride-rich lipoproteins from the plasma. This is probably mediated by an increase in lipoprotein lipase activity.

A common occurrence with plasma triglyceride reduction in general, but which is especially evident with gemfibrozil use, is an increase in plasma LDL-C levels concomitant with the triglyceride (VLDL-C) lowering. Whether this truly represents an increased atherosclerotic risk is uncertain. The increased levels of HDL-C noted with gemfibrozil use have been shown by HDL-C turnover studies to represent a highly active reverse transport particle (as is shown for probucol).

Clinical Use

Gemfibrozil is currently available in 600 mg capsules with a usual dose of one capsule taken twice daily. It should be regarded as the drug of choice for all hypertriglyceridemic conditions (IIb, III, IV and V).

The clinician should take note that VLDL-C-lowering can cause a reciprocal increase in LDL-C values, especially at higher levels of hypertriglyceridemia. However, this effect can readily be countered with the addition of a bile acid sequestrant.

In general, in patients with lesser degrees of hypertriglyceridemia, a 15 to 20 percent plasma LDL-C reduction is noted.

Gemfibrozil causes few side effects unless used in combination with HMG-CoA reductase inhibitors. The risk of myositis from this combined modality should relatively contraindicate this combination.

Gemfibrozil causes a predictable decline of plasma triglyceride (VLDL-C) levels with an increase in plasma HDL-C in virtually all patients with hypertriglyceridemia. The magnitude of this effect is directly related to the degree of hypertriglyceridemia. Generally, a 30 to 60 percent triglyceride reduction is noted, with a concomitant rise of plasma HDL-C levels of 15 to 20 percent.

Because of the relatively few clinical side effects noted with this medication, clinical monitoring considerations are notably fewer than for other medications. Nevertheless, these should include serial liver function studies.

The use of gemfibrozil for the treatment of secondary dyslipidemia associated with diabetes mellitus (hypertriglyceridemia) is suggested, especially because of its HDL-C-raising effects. Also other plasma triglyceride-lowering medications (niacin and omega-3 fatty acids) can worsen glycemic control.

Side Effects

Possible side effects from use of fibric acid derivatives may include:

- Gastrointestinal complaints (occurring in three to five percent of patients):
  - Abdominal pain
  - Diarrhea
  - Nausea
- Liver function study changes, including:
  - Rises in transaminase
  - Declines in phosphatase

Muscle tenderness should raise the suspicion of myositis, which requires CPK determination. The incidence of this disorder is increased with concomitant use of HMG-CoA reductase inhibitors.

Gemfibrozil can increase the effects of oral anticoagulants.

Increased biliary lithogenicity potentially results in increased occurrence of gallstones.

Possible side effects and use of clofibrate are discussed in Section #16.

Other Fibric Acid Agents

Although gemfibrozil and clofibrate are the only currently available therapeutic agents in the United States, other fibric acid derivatives are in development and some are currently available in certain other countries. These include:

- Benzafibrate
- Fenofibrate
- Ciprofibrate
- Etofibrate

Compared with clofibrate, these compounds are more effective in plasma LDL-C lowering (almost twice as great in Type IIa subjects), but they have a lesser triglyceride lowering and plasma HDL-C-raising effect than gemfibrozil.

These drugs have not yet been subjected to large-scale, long-term, placebo-controlled trials. Thus, available long-term data are generally based on uncontrolled observations. However, it is worth noting that clinical information from 15 years of open label experience is available involving over 3,500 subjects who received fenofibrate.

Although fenofibrate is not yet approved by the FDA, it is currently available by prescription in Europe, given as a 300 mg/day dose. Besides its effect in lipoprotein lipase-mediated reductions in plasma triglycerides, fenofibrate appears to cause an HMG-CoA reductase inhibitory suppression of cholesterol synthesis. This may affect an increase in hepatic LDL-C receptors, possibly accounting for its effect in plasma LDL-C lowering.

References

Hunninghake DB, Peters JR: Effects of fibric acid derivatives on blood lipid and lipoprotein levels. Am J Med 1987;83(Suppl 5B):44.

Kesaniemi YA, Grundy SM: Influence of gemfibrozil and clofibrate on metabolism of cholesterol and plasma triglycerides in man. JAMA 1984; 251:2241.

Leaf DA, Connor WE, et al: The hypolipemic effects of gemfibrozil in Type V hyperlipidemia. A double-blind, crossover study. JAMA 1989; 262:3154.

Lewis JE: Clinical use of gemfibrozil: a controlled multicentre trial. Practical Cardiology 1983;9:99.

Magarian GJ, Lucas LM, Colley C: Gemfibrozil-induced myopathy. Arch Intern Med 1991;151:1873.

Mannien V, Elo O, Frick H, et al: Lipid alterations and decline in the incidence of coronary heart disease in the Helsinki Heart Study. JAMA 1988;260:641.

Saku K, Gartside PS, et al: Mechanism of action of gemfibrozil on lipoprotein metabolism. J Clin Invest 1985;75:1702.

NOTES

#13 HMG-CoA Reductase Inhibitors

Clinical Information

A new class of inhibitors of the rate-limiting enzyme in cholesterol biosynthesis (HMG-CoA reductase) represents a recently developed group of potent LDL-C-lowering medications. These compounds include:

- Lovastatin (Mevacor®)
- Simvastatin (Zocor®)
- Mevastatin (Compactin®)
- Pravastatin (Eptastatin®)
- Fluvastatin

Lovastatin has been the most widely available for general use, and is presented as the prototype.

The results of current clinical trials make these the medications of choice for the heterozygotic form of familial hypercholesterolemia. They are an attractive alternative to the bile sequestrants as a first-line agent for other forms of hypercholesterolemia because they are easily taken. However, they should always be used with careful attention paid to potential side effects.

Mode of Action

As previously stated, these compounds act as competitive inhibitors of cholesterol biosynthesis involving the rate-limiting enzyme to cholesterol production (HMG-CoA reductase). In polygenic forms of hypercholesterolemia, this effect causes a marked lowering of plasma LDL-C levels (24 to 40 percent) as LDL particle synthesis is reduced and LDL particle clearance is also increased.

Because the cellular cholesterol depletion caused by these agents stimulates increased LDL particle receptor activity, an ultimate LDL-C-lowering effect is induced by receptor up-regulation. This receptor-mediated LDL-C-lowering effect is especially important in heterozygotic forms of familial hypercholesterolemia. The medication also has a small, but significant, HDL-C-raising (6.6 to 9.5 percent) and triglyceride-lowering (10 to 19 percent) effect.

Clinical Use

Lovastatin (Mevacor®) can be given in initial oral doses of 20 mg QPM or with the evening meal. This can be advanced to a maximum dose of 40 mg BID with an anticipated dose related LDL-C reduction. These amounts can also be given as a once-a-day dose. Because the majority of cholesterol synthesis occurs in the body at night, single-dose plasma cholesterol-lowering regimens are best given as an HS dose.

The anticipated plasma LDL-C-lowering effect from HMG-CoA reductase inhibitor medications can approach 40 percent in patients with familial hypercholesterolemia. This class of medications can treat all forms of hypercholesterolemia, including:

- Familial
- Polygenic
- Familial combined dyslipidemia

In familial combined dyslipidemia, HMG-CoA reductase inhibitors are an effective first-line medication for patients with a phenotypic IIA pattern especially for those with documented evidence of severe CAD. Lovastatin has also been shown effective in treating hypercholesterolemia associated with mild triglyceride elevations (ie, phenotype IIB). Patients not responding (compliance issues included) to bile acid sequestrant therapy can be expeditiously changed to this category of medication.

Side Effects

The incidence of side effects after one year of use has been evaluated for lovastatin at various doses in a placebo-controlled intervention (EXCEL) study. A very low incidence of adverse side effects was present. In particular, at 20 mg BID:

- Transaminase elevation (>3x upper limit Normal)=0.9 percent, increasing with dose increase
- Muscle symptoms with any level of CPK elevation = 1.6 percent (not different from placebo)
- No apparent risk of lenticular opacity formation (previously advocated ophthalmological slit lamp evaluation has been dropped)

The major clinical issue for use of these medications involves potential hepatotoxicity. Liver function tests should be obtained at baseline, with follow-ups every four to six weeks for the first 15 months of therapy and less frequently thereafter. Transaminase levels increasing threefold above normal upper limits require discontinuation of the medication. Active liver disease is a contraindication to HMG-CoA reductase inhibitor.

Myopathy, which can occur with medication use, is most frequently noted with the concomitant use of:

- Immunosuppressive therapy
- Fibric acid derivatives
- Lipid-lowering doses of niacin

Rhabdomyalysis may precipitate acute renal failure. Thus, these medication combinations become relatively contraindicated. Recently a 5 mg strength lovastatin has been released as a low dose which could be employed in this setting. Similarly, concomitant use with coumadin may prolong the prothrombin time and potentiate bleeding risk.

HMG-CoA reductase inhibitors should not be used during pregnancy or before 20 years of age.

General side effects include:

- Changes in bowel habits
- Nausea
- Headaches
- Fatigue
- Insomnia
- Skin rashes

These side effects were not prominent in the EXCEL study, but should be recognized since they were suggested by other clinical studies.

As discussed in Section #1, evidence from the FATS showed a greater regression in CAD lesions with lovastatin than conventional therapy. A lupus-like syndrome associated with lovastatin has been reported. The currently available findings indicate that lovastatin is a generally safe and effective medication, however; the long term effects of medications which impair cholesterol synthesis are unknown. Currently large-scale CAD reducing intervention trials are underway which will continue to demonstrate the safety and role of this medication.

Other HMG-CoA Reductase Inhibitors

Although lovastatin has been the most widely available compound with the most extensive clinical study, other HMG-CoA reductase inhibitors are available internationally, and have been recently approved for use in the United States including:

- Pravastatin (Eptastatin – Bristol Myers-Squibb)
- Simvastatin (Zocar – Merck Sharpe and Dohne)

These will be considered in comparison with lovastatin, the prototype compound of this class previously discussed.

Pravastatin

Pravastatin is a hydrophylic compound which may minimize its CNS effects. It is administered as an active lactone ring which is hydrolyzed to inactive metabolites by the liver. This may increase its tissue specificity to the liver and minimize potential systemic effects.

Pravastatin has a major effect of dose response LDL-C lowering as dose increases from 5 to 40 mg/day. The dose range is 10 to 40 mg/day in single or divided doses. An LDL-C and Apo-B lowering by approximately 30 percent is typically experienced. Lesser effects are noted in triglyceride lowering (approximately 15 percent) and HDL-C raising (approximately 10 percent).

The clinical indications for the use of pravastatin mirror those of lovastatin, ie, in patients with hypercholesterolemia, especially familial hypercholesterolemia and for most phenotype IIA particularly with established CAD.

Similarly, pravastatin appears to have a comparable adverse risk profile to other U.S. approved agents as shown by double-blind randomized placebo control trials in the U.S. and abroad. An Italian multicenter study of 385 primary hypercholesterolemics randomly assigned to provastatin 40 mg/HS or Gemfibrozil 600 mg BID for 24 weeks showed a very low incidence of side effects which was similar for both medications. Major issues include potential hepatotoxicity, skin rashes and headaches which are reversible. Again, the long term experience with this medication is relatively limited compared with lovastatin.

Simvastatin

Simvastatin, an analog of lovastatin, also administered as a hydrophobic lactone and hydrolized in the liver to its active form. Simvastatin has a similar effect on lipoprotein profiles as the other compounds in this class. A major LDL-C lowering effect of up to 50 percent has been shown in Familial Hypercholesterolemics. A potential advantage of this compound is the lower dosage and frequency of administration when compared with other HMG-CoA reductase inhibitors. Clinical trials with simvastatin are more limited than those for lovastatin, although simvastatin has enjoyed some commerical use outside of the U.S. with an apparent adverse side-effect profile similar to other compounds of this group.

References

Ahmad S: Lovastatin induced lupus erythematosus. Arch Intern Med 1991;151:1667.

Alberts AW: HMG-CoA reductase inhibitors – the development. Atheroscler Rev 1988;18:123.

EXCEL: Expanded Clinical Evaluation of Lovastatin (EXCEL) study results. Arch Intern Med 1991;151:43.

Hoeg JM, et al: Effectiveness of Mevinolin on plasma lipoprotein concentrations in Type II hyperlipoproteinemia. Am J Cardiol 1986;57:933.

Hunninglake DB, Knopp RH, Schonfeld G, et al: Efficacy and safety of pravastatin in patients with primary hypercholesterolemia I. A dose response study. Atherosclerosis 1990;85:81.

Illingworth DR: Comparative efficacy of once versus twice daily Mevinolin in the therapy of familial hypercholesterolemia. Clin Pharmacol Ther 1986;40:338.

Illingworth DR, Brown SP, Larsen KK: Long-term experience with HMG-CoA reductase inhibitors in the therapy of hypercholesterolemia. Atheroscler Rev 1988;18:161.

The Italian Multicenter Pravastatin Study I. Pravastatin vs. gemfibrozil in the treatment of primary hypercholesterolemia. Arch Intern Med 1990;151:146.

Jones PH, Farmer JA, Cressman MD, et al: Once daily pravastatin in patients with primary hypercholesterolemia: A dose response study. Clin Cardiol 1991;14:146.

Moseley ST, Kalinowaki SS, Schafer BL, et al: Tissue-selective acute effects of inhibitors of 3-hydroxy-3-methylglutaryl co-enzmye. A reductase on cholesterol biosynthesis in the lens. J Lipid Res 1989;30:1411.

O'Connor P, et al: BMJ 1990;300:667.

Pan HY, DeVault AR, Wang-Iverson D: Comparative pharmacokinetic and pharmacodynamics of pravastatin and lovastatin. J Clin Pharmacol 1990;30:1128.

The Lovastatin Study Group II. Therapeutic response to lovastatin (Mevinolin) in nonfamilial hypercholesterolemia: a multicenter study. JAMA 1986;267:2829.

Reihner E, Rudling M, Stahlberg D, et al: Influence of pravastatin, a specific inhibitor of HMG-CoA reductase, on hepatic metabolism of cholesterol. N Engl J Med 1990;323:224.

Stein E, Kreisberg R, Miller V, et al: Effects of simvastatin and cholestyramine in familial and nonfamilial hypercholesterolemia. Arch Intern Med 1990;150:341.

Symposium. Simvastatin: A once-a-day treatment for hypercholesterolemia. Am J Med 1989;87(4A):1S.

Vega GL, Grundy SM: Management of primary mixed hyperlipidemia with lovastatin. Arch Intern Med 1990;150:1313.

Ytre-Arne K, Nordoy A: Simvastatin and cholestyramine in the long-term treatment of hypercholesterolemia. J Intern Med 1989;226:285.

NOTES

#14 Probucol

Clinical Information

Probucol (Lorelco®) represents a unique medication that:

- Appears to reduce atherogenesis by preventing the oxidative modification of LDL-C to its more atherogenic form
- Has a plasma LDL-C-lowering effect of lesser magnitude than either:
  - Bile acid sequestrants
  - HMG-CoA reductase inhibitors
- Is suggested as a second-line medication for the treatment of hypercholesterolemias

Mode of Action

Probucol lowers both plasma LDL-C and HDL-C levels by mechanisms that are not altogether certain. The plasma LDL-C-lowering effect appears to result from both:

- Increased LDL-C catabolism
- Increased biliary cholesterol excretion

Increased LDL-C removal appears to involve non-LDL-C receptor pathways; therefore, this medication is useful in treating homozygous familial hypercholesterolemia.

More recently, probucol has been shown to reduce the oxidative modification of LDL-C that occurs in arterial endothelial cells. This oxidative effect causes LDL-C modification and is indicated to promote atherosclerosis by increasing mon-

14.

ocyte/macrophage and smooth muscle cell cholesterol uptake. This effect promotes endothelial cell injury, leading to atherogenesis. This important antioxidant effect of probucol on LDL oxidation may explain its effect in reducing the progression of atherosclerosis in the Watanabe rabbit model.

The cause of reduced plasma HDL-C levels occurring with probucol administration is not certain but does not necessarily indicate a deleterious effect. Current evidence indicates that, although probucol may lower total plasma HDL-C levels, the kind of HDL-C produced is actually a more rapidly turning-over particle.

In this sense this HDL-C level is not necessarily pathological and may actually represent a "healthier" antiatherogenic form of HDL-C with increased reverse transport capabilities.

Clinical Use

Probucol can be used for all primary forms of hypercholesterolemia, but based on current evidence, it is best used as a secondary line of therapy. An eight to 15 percent reduction of plasma LDL-C levels should be anticipated, with a concomitant 15 to 20 percent plasma HDL-C lowering.

Probucol is given as a 500 mg BID dose. This medication is generally well tolerated, with side effects occurring in less than 10 percent of all patients. EKG tracings should be monitored during therapy because of the QT interval prolongation, which is occasionally induced.

The Probucol Quantitative Regression Sweden Trial (PQRST), is an ongoing three year, double-blind randomized trial designed to determine whether probucol can retard or regress atherosclerosis in hypercholesterolemics. The results of the trial (which is projected to conclude in December 1992) will provide important clinical information regarding this medication.

Side Effects

Possible side effects resulting from use of probucol may include:

- Diarrhea
- Flatulence
- Abdominal pain
- Nausea
- Hyperhidrosis
- Fetid sweat
- Angioneurotic edema
- Prolongation of the QT interval on EKG, which, however, has not been shown to cause arrhythmias in humans

References

Kita K, Nagano Y, Yokode M, et al: Probucol prevents progression of atherosclerosis in the Watanabe heritable hyperlipemic rabbit. Proc Natl Acad Sci USA. 1987;84:5928.

Mellies MJ, Gartside PS, Galtfeleter L, Glueck GJ: Effect of probucol on plasma cholesterol high and low density lipoprotein cholesterol and apolipoprotein A_1 and A_2 in adults with primary familial hypercholesterolemia. Metabolism 1980;20:956.

Nestel PJ, Billington T: Effects of probucol on low density lipoprotein removal and high density lipoprotein synthesis. Atherosclerosis 1981;38:203.

Symposium: New developments in the treatment of hypercholesterlemia – probucol. Am J Cardiol 1986;57:1H.

Walltius G, Carlson LA, Erikson V, et al: Development of femoral atherosclerosis in hypercholesterlemic patients during treatment with cholestyramine and probucol/placebo. Probucol Quantitative Regression Sweden Trial. A status report. Am J Cardiol 1988;62:37B.

CENTER

INDEX

#15 Omega-3 Fatty Acids (Fish Oil)

Clinical Information

Omega-3 fatty acids are a class of polyunsaturated fatty acids primarily found in marine oils. Produced by phytoplankton and algae, they accumulate in fish as they ascend the biological food chain. Since initial epidemiological studies of the Greenland Eskimos indicated omega-3 fatty acid intake may be protective against CAD, a great deal of research interest has been expended in identifying the mechanism(s) of this potential protection.

The two biologically important omega-3 fatty acids used in commercial preparations are:

- Eicosapentaenoic acid (EPA), C20:5
- Docosahexaenoic acid (DHA), C22:6

Although pharmaceutical doses of these fatty acids (4.5 grams/day) can be effective in lowering plasma triglycerides, the effects of omega-3 fatty acids on plasma lipoproteins are less consistent with lesser doses and have variable effects, depending upon the underlying lipid disorder. In addition, the use of omega-3 fatty acids may provide unwanted calories (nine kcal/gram) and is contraindicated in persons who have bleeding disorders or take anticoagulants.

Mode of Action

Omega-3 fatty acids have a profound effect in lowering plasma triglycerides by reducing hepatic VLDL production, which may require doses of 10 to 20 grams per day.

Omega-3 fatty acids also increase peripheral utilization of plasma VLDL. A lack of consistent effects on plasma HDL-C levels is apparent. Reports indicate that in certain lipid disorders (phenotype IV and IIb), omega-3 fatty acids tend to raise plasma LDL-C levels, an effect also noted with fibric acid derivatives. This likely reflects the result of increased catabolism of VLDL precursor particles, and results in increased plasma levels of apolipoprotein B. This effect is not noted in patients with the IIa phenotype. Alternatively, recent reports indicate that the saturated fat and cholesterol content which varies in different commercial preparations can effect the LDL-C response.

The atherogenic significance of these findings is uncertain. A current review (Harris) of the available clinical trials involving the effects of omega-3 fatty acids on plasma lipids and lipoproteins emphasizes the heterogeneous nature of the methods involved in these trials, rendering their collective interpretation difficult. A more recently published clinical experience from one group (Davidson) shows the effects of fish oil capsule supplementation on patients with different dislipidemias.

Possibly, the potential beneficial effects of omega-3 fatty acids with respect to CAD risk are not only mediated by plasma lipoprotein metabolism but also involve arterial eicosanoid metabolism. Arachidonic acid (C20:5, omega-6), found in platelets and the blood vessel endothelium, is converted by a series of transformations to metabolically active prostanoid metabolites. Thromboxane A_2, produced by thromboxane synthetase in platelets, causes vasoconstriction and enhancement of platelet aggregation. Prostacyclin synthetase produces prostacyclin (PGI_2) from endothelium-derived prostanoid metabolites. PGI_2 causes vasodilatation and inhibits platelet aggregation.

EPA can effect these metabolic pathways, which influence the thrombotic aspects of the thrombo-atherogenic process by substituting as a precursor metabolite for arachidonic acid to form thromboxane A_3, and PGI_3 creates a less thrombogenic milieu. This may explain the reduction in thrombo-atherogenic findings occurring with omega-3 fatty acid supplementation in animal studies.

Clinical Uses

A broad array of "fish oil capsules" are available commercially. It is important to recognize that these vary in terms of the fatty acid and cholesterol content. These preparations also are available as the triglyceride, the ethyl and the methyl forms of the omega-3 fatty acids all of which appear to be well utilized by the body. They can be considered as therapeutic to severe hypertriglyceridemia (Types IV and V) and less severe forms (IIb) not responding to other therapeutic agents (Davidson). It should be noted that this form of therapy is inexpensive relative to currently available pharmaceutics but is not typically covered by most health insurance policies, hemostatic monitoring is suggested.

Alternatively, the current evidence of the optimal dose of omega-3 fatty acid for reducing CAD risk is suggested by findings in a population of 835 men in the Netherlands. This study suggested that men who consumed an average of two fish meals a week (or 30 grams of fish daily) had a significant reduction of CAD events over a 20-year period compared with non-fish eaters.

A more recent, randomized, controlled dietary trial resulted in a significant reduction (29 percent) in two-year, all-cause mortality for the men consuming increased fish intake. This trial assigned 2,033 post-MI men to dietary study groups of:

- Two fish meals per week
- A low-fat diet
- A high-fiber diet

This outcome was not apparent in the other dietary groups and suggests that CAD-lowering benefits can occur at markedly lower amounts of omega-3 fatty acid intake than are characteristic of the Eskimo diet, and are insufficient to influence plasma lipid levels.

Given these findings, the health practitioner should probably encourage the consumption of increased fish meals as there is currently no evidence to provide direct support for the use of fish oil capsules for reducing CAD risk. Further investigation to assess the long-term safety and efficacy of marine oil is needed before widespread use is recommended. Table 15.1 provides a list of amounts of EPA and DHA in various supplements and foods.

TABLE 15.1 – **Amount of Omega-3 Fatty Acids (EPA and DHA) in Fish Oil Supplements and Selected Fish and Seafoods**

Food	**EPA (g/100 g of food)**	**DHA (g/100 g of food)**
Cod liver oil	9.0	9.5
Max EPA	7.1	4.3
Anchovy	0.5	0.9
Bass, fresh water	0.1	0.2
Catfish, channel	0.1	0.2
Haddock	0.1	0.1
Halibut, Pacific	0.7	0.9
Herring, Atlantic	0.7	0.9
Mackerel, Atlantic	0.9	1.0
Perch	0.1	0.1
Salmon, chinook	0.8	0.6
Salmon, pink	0.4	0.6
Smelt	0.1	0.2
Sturgeon, Atlantic	1.0	0.5
Trout, rainbow	0.1	0.4
Tuna, albacore	0.3	1.0
Crab, dungeness	0.2	0.1
Lobster	0.1	0.1
Shrimp	0.2	0.2
Octopus	0.1	0.1
Oyster	0.2	0.2
Scallop	0.1	0.1

Side Effects

- Increased bleeding tendency (contraindication for patients with bleeding disorders or who take anticoagulants)
- Increased caloric intake
- Vitamin A and D toxicity when fish liver oil is taken in excessive amounts
- Theoretical possibility of causing vitamin E deficiency by increasing polyunsaturated fat intake
- Potential effects in pregnancy are unclear
- Can aggravate glycemic control in non-insulin-dependent diabetes

References

Burr ML, Gilbert JF, et al: Effects of changes of fat, fish, and fibre intakes on death and myocardial reinfarction: diet and reinfarction trial (DART). Lancet 1989;2:757.

Davidson MH, Burns JH, Subbaiah PV, et al: Marine oil capsule therapy for the treatment of hyperlipidemia. Arch Intern Med 1991;151:1732.

Harris WS: Fish oils and plasma lipid and lipoprotein metabolism in humans: a critical review. J Lipid Research 1989;30:785.

Harris WS, Connor WE, et al: Dietary omega-3 fatty acids prevent carbohydrate-induced hypertriglyceridemia. Metabolism 1984;33:1016.

Harris WS, Zucker ML, Dvjovne CA: Omega-3 fatty acids in hypertriglyceridemic patients: triglycerides vs. methyl esters. Am J Clin Nutr 1988;48:992.

Kromhout D, Bosschieter EB, de Lezenne Coulander C: The inverse relationship between fish consumption and 20-year mortality from coronary heart disease. N Engl J Med 1985;312:1205.

Glauber H, Wallace P, et al: Adverse metabolism effect of omega-3 fatty acids in non-insulin-dependent diabetes mellitus. Ann Intern Med 1988;108:663.

Goodnight SH Jr, Harris WS, et al: Polyunsaturated fatty acids, hyperlipidemia and thrombosis. Arteriosclerosis 1982;2:87.

Leaf DA: Omega-3 fatty acids and coronary artery disease, more than a fish tale. Postgrad Med 1989;85:237.

NOTES

#16 Secondary-Line Medications

Clofibrate (Atromid-S®)

Although clofibrate (Atromid-S®) has been shown to be effective in reducing plasma lipids and lowering long-term incidence of CAD, the concomitantly increased incidence of non-cardiological mortality (malignant neoplasms, particularly of the gastrointestinal tract, and cholecystitis) has limited its use. Gemfibrozil should be used as a safer alternative.

Current findings indicate that clofibrate should be restricted to treatment of Type III and Type IV dyslipidemias unresponsive to diet and other medications.

Neomycin

A nonabsorbable aminoglycoside antibiotic with hypocholesterolemic effects, this medication is limited by side effects of:

- Diarrhea and abdominal cramps in 30 percent of patients
- Ototoxicity
- Nephrotoxicity

This medication should be considered outmoded.

d-Thyroxine

d-Thyroxine lowers LDL-C by stimulating LDL-C receptor activity but can cause:

- Cardiac arrhythmias
- Nervousness

- Increased sweating
- Tremors

16.

This medication is best used only to treat dyslipidemia that has occurred secondary to hypothyroidism.

References

Coronary Drug Project: Findings leading to further modifications of its protocol with respect to dextrothyroxine. JAMA 1972;220:996.

Coronary Drug Project: Clofibrate and niacin in coronary heart disease. JAMA 1975;231:360.

Committee of Principal Investigators: A cooperative trial in primary prevention of ischemic heart disease using clofibrate. Br Heart J 1978;40:1069.

Samuel P: Treatment of hypercholesterolemia with neomycin: a time for reappraisal. N Engl J Med 1979;301:595.

#17 Combination Therapies

Introduction

The purpose of combination therapy is to improve lipid-lowering effects to achieve therapeutic levels. This is best done by using medications that have different mechanisms of action and whose simultaneous use does not cause untoward side effects. A number of potential combination therapies exist. Presented here are a few potential combinations involving double therapies. Triple therapies also exist.

LDL-C Lowering

- Bile acid sequestrant plus HMG-CoA reductase inhibitor
- HMG-CoA reductase inhibitor plus probucol (especially for familial hypercholesterolemia due to the receptor-independent pathway mechanism of probucol)
- Bile acid sequestrant plus niacin
- Bile acid sequestrant plus probucol
- Guar gum and gemfibrozil

VLDL-C Lowering

- Bile acid sequestrant plus niacin (for Type IIb phenotype, currently more effectively managed with gemfibrozil alone)
- Bile acid sequestrant plus gemfibrozil
- Gemfibrozil and niacin

Contraindicated Combination

Relative contraindication is encountered with HMG-CoA reductase inhibitor plus gemfibrozil, which causes increased incidence of myositis.

17.

References

Dvjovne CA, Krehbiel P, et al: Probucol with colestipol in the treatment of hypercholesterolemia. Ann Intern Med 1983;100:477.

Illingworth DR: Mevinolin plus colestipol of therapy for severe heterozygous familial hypercholesterolemia. Ann Intern Med 1984;101:598.

Illingworth DR, et al: Colestipol plus nicotinic acid in treatment of heterozygous familial hypercholesterolamia. Lancet 1981;1:296.

Kuo PT, Kostis JB, et al: Familial type II hyperlipoproteinemia with coronary heart disease: effect of colestipol plus nicotinic acid. Chest 1981;79:286.

Tuomilehto J, Silvasti M, et al: Guar gum and gemfibrozil – an effective combination in the treatment of hypercholesterolemia. Atherosclerosis 1989;76:71.

#18 Therapeutic Goals

Hypercholesterolemia

Ideally, LDL-C should be reduced to less than 130 mg% (3.4 mmol/L), especially in the setting of two or more CAD risk factors. Based on the recent findings from regression studies cited in Section #1, the most appropriate target for patients with established CAD is an LDL-C below 100 mg% (2.6 mmol/L). For patients without evidence of increased CAD risk, a plasma LDL-C target level can be 160 mg% (4.1 mmol/L) or less.

Hypertriglyceridemia

Plasma triglycerides should be below 150 mg% (1.7 mmol/L). Plasma triglyceride lowering in the hypertriglyceridemic patient typically has a secondary benefit of raising plasma HDL-C levels and is especially important in patients with familial combined dyslipidemia, dysbetalipoproteinemia (type III), or those who provide a strong family tendency for CAD. However, when this goal is not realistic in the setting of severe hypertriglyceridemia, a target goal of maintaining plasma triglyceride levels below 500 mg% (5.6 mmol/L) is warranted to reduce the risk for pancreatitis, although in this case many practitioners will settle for the best outcome achievable.

References

The Expert Panel: Report of the National Cholesterol Education Program Expert Panel on detection, evaluation and treatment of high blood cholesterol in adults. Arch Intern Med 1988;148:36.

NOTES

18.

#19 Intervention Guidelines: United States/Eureopean

Screening

The National Cholesterol Education Program Adult Treatment Panel has established screening and therapeutic guidelines for all adults over 20 years of age. Total plasma cholesterol values are used as an initial screening measurement, as shown in Table 19.1. A value below 200 mg% (5.2 mmol/L) is considered to be desirable, whereas a value exceeding 240 mg% (6.2 mmol/L) becomes potentially high risk, requiring further assessment.

For patients with desirable plasma cholesterol levels, the principles of a prudent diet (low fat, low cholesterol) should be provided. Repeat cholesterol values will not be needed for another five years.

High risk status requiring further evaluation is achieved when the borderline-high plasma cholesterol is in the 200 to 239 mg% range in the presence of definite CAD or two or more of the following risk factors:

- Male gender
- Family history of premature CAD before 55 years of age
- Cigarette smoking
- Hypertension
- Diabetes mellitus
- Obesity (at least 30 percent overweight)

For those in the 200 to 239 mg% range who are not of high-risk status, Step 1 dietary advice should be given, with a follow-up cholesterol determination obtained after one year.

For patients identified as potentially high risk, a fasting plasma lipoprotein analysis is required for further diagnostic considerations. These considerations are based on the need to obtain the level of plasma LDL-C.

A scheme similar to that used in assessing total plasma cholesterol level is employed for plasma LDL-C values, as shown in Table 19.2. If plasma LDL-C level is below 130 mg% (3.4 mmol/L), the patient should be considered to be at a desirable cholesterol level. A borderline LDL-C level (130 to 159 mg% [3.4 to 4.1 mmol/L]) without the presence of CAD or two or more CAD risk factors should receive Step 1 dietary advice and an annual follow-up determination of plasma cholesterol.

The remaining patients (having LDL equal to or greater than 160 mg% (4.1 mmol/L), or 130 to 159 mg% (3.4 to 4.1 mmol/L) with definite CAD or two or more CAD risk factors) should be screened for possible secondary causes of dyslipidemia, as described in Section #7. These patients should be initiated on Step 1 dietary intervention with six-week follow-up determinations of plasma LDL-C to assess therapeutic response.

Although these recommendations are criticized as not relevant for all individual cases and for not considering plasma HDL-C levels, it must be recognized that because they are designed for population level intervention, certain individuals may not be effectively dealt with by these guidelines. However, because these are public health-directed approaches, they provide the most appropriate advice with respect to detection and treatment of hypercholesterolemia.

Further issues in interpreting plasma HDL-C levels are discussed in Section #1.

Although these guidelines appear to ignore plasma HDL-C, this is not entirely true; a plasma HDL-C level less than 35 mg% (0.9 mmol/L) is counted as a CAD risk factor. In addition, plasma HDL-C levels are accounted for indirectly in the determination of plasma LDL-C levels calculated by subtracting plasma HDL-C levels from total plasma cholesterol. Thus, a low plasma HDL-C level is indirectly reflected as an increased CAD risk setting by virtue of an increased plasma LDL-C value at any level of total plasma cholesterol.

In addition, targeting LDL-C appears warranted based on the low incidence of CAD events in non-Western cultures, where individuals consume relatively little fat. Although these individuals have typically low plasma LDL-C and HDL-C levels, the lack of CAD in these populations is probably best ascribed to low plasma LDL-C levels.

It may be only in Western cultures, where a high dietary fat intake is the norm, that increased plasma HDL-C values are of anti-atherogenic significance. Based on this concept, it could be argued that, if plasma LDL-C levels were appropriately reduced, plasma HDL-C levels would be of less importance.

Conversely, evidence from major clinical trials conducted in industrialized countries emphasizes the importance of plasma HDL-C levels as a CAD risk factor when plasma cholesterol levels are below 200 mg% (5.2 mmol/L).

A practical reason for targeting plasma LDL-C for intervention strategies is that, in contrast to the number of hygienic and drug interventions available to lower plasma LDL-C levels, there are currently few interventions available for effectively raising plasma HDL-C levels. In addition, intervention studies aimed at HDL-C lowering also influence other lipoproteins. Therefore, a "pure" interpretation is difficult. On the other hand, the POSCH has shown that isolated LDL-C lowering by partial bypass reduced CAD risk in patients with familial hypercholesterolemia.

Treatment

Because the goal of treatment is to reduce mean plasma cholesterol levels, it is advisable to:

- Achieve desirable body weight levels
- Participate regularly in physical activity
- Consume a diet that is:
  - Low in saturated fats and cholesterol
  - High in complex carbohydrates and dietary fiber

Specific guidelines are developed for dietary treatment of high-risk patients identified with elevated plasma LDL-C levels greater than:

- 160 mg% (4.1 mmol/L)
- 130 mg% (3.4 mmol/L) in the presence of:
  - CAD
  - Two or more CAD risk factors

Table 19.3 provides a general summary of the dietary guidelines aimed at lowering the plasma LDL-C levels.

Step 1 advice can be initiated by a physician with follow-up determination of fasting plasma LDL-C levels measured on a six-week basis to assess therapeutic response. A three to four week period of time is generally needed to assess the effects of any plasma lipid interventions.

The goal is to lower plasma LDL-C below 130 mg% (3.4 mmol/L) when CAD or two or more CAD risk factors are present or below 160 mg% (4.1 mmol/L) when these conditions do not exist. Again, the findings from regression studies published since the 1988 Expert Panel Guidelines (discussed in Section #1) suggest a goal of LDL-C lowering below 100 mg% (2.6 mmol/L) is indicated in the setting of established CAD. If this outcome does not occur after 12 weeks of Step 1 dietary intervention, the patient should be referred for dietary counseling for another six week trial of the Step 1 diet.

If the LDL-C goal is not achieved at this point, the Step 2 diet should be attempted. A total of six months of dietary measures is suggested before considering pharmaceutical intervention. See Sections #20 and #21 for a description of the specific components of the dietary guidelines. The rationale for pharmaceutical intervention is described Section #8.

Due to the limited scope of this manual, it is advisable that more extensive reading of nutrition-related material be done in order for the practitioner to be able to provide comprehensive dietary management.

TABLE 19.1 – **Total Plasma Cholesterol Levels and CAD Risk**

HIGH –

- Total plasma cholesterol ≥ 240 mg%
- Total plasma cholesterol 200 to 239 mg% in the presence of CAD or 2 or more CAD risk factors

BORDERLINE –

- Total plasma cholesterol 200 to 239 mg% without CAD or 2 or more CAD risk factors

DESIRABLE –

- Total plasma cholesterol ≤ 200 mg%

TABLE 19.2 – **Plasma LDL-C Levels and CAD Risk**

HIGH –

- Plasma LDL-C ≥ 160 mg%
- Plasma LDL-C 130 to 159 mg% in the presence of CAD or 2 or more CAD risk factors

BORDERLINE –

- Plasma LDL-C 130 to 159 mg% without CAD or 2 or more CAD risk factors

DESIRABLE –

- Plasma LDL-C ≤ 130 mg%*

***Note**: Evidence from current regression studies supports lowering LDL-C ≤ 100 mg% in the setting of established CAD.

TABLE 19.3 – **Dietary Guidelines**

	Percent of Dietary Calories	
	Step 1	**Step 2**
Saturated fat	< 10%	< 7%
Polyunsaturated fat	< 10%	< 10%
Monounsaturated fat	10 to 15%	10 to 15 %
Total fat	< 30%	< 30%
Carbohydrates	50 to 60%	50 to 60%
Protein	10 to 20%	10 to 20%
Cholesterol	< 300 mg/d	< 200 mg/d

European Guidelines

The European guidelines for detection and treatment of lipid disorders differs from the standards suggested for North America (United States and Canada). In addition, certain lipid lowering medications are commercially available in European countries which are not currently in prescribed use in North America. Because the units of measurement of plasma cholesterol and triglyceride levels typically employed outside of the United States (mg% or mg/dl) are expressed in mmoles/liter (mmol/L), Table 19.4 is provided to serve as reference which supplies conversion factors between measurements expressed according to these systems. Mmol/L represents the Systeme Internationale (SI) units which are the Internationally recognized nomenclature system generally used in medical literature and should be learned by recalcitrant health care practitioners of all nations. SI units have been provided in parenthesis throughout this text.

The guidelines of the European Atherosclerosis Society (EAS) are similar to their North American counterparts, and are essentially comparable because of the basis of their common mission. The purpose of this section is to delineate any existing major differences rather than to reiterate all of their similarities. The reader who wishes to read the original EAS report will find its overall content to be generally the same as the North American guidelines (ie, National Cholesterol Education Panel), although some differences in the clinical approach are apparent. The EAS similarly suggests LDL-C lowering with the goal of 135 mg% (3.5 mmol/L) in high risk and 155 mg% (4.0 mmol/L) in low risk individuals. The risk of pancreatitis provides the rationale for the therapeutic goal in managing severe hypertriglycerdemia; suggested plasma triglyceride levels are below 1,000 mg% (11 mmol/L), with an optimal level of less than 500 mg% (5.6 mmol/L). These therapeutic goals are similar to those recommended by the National Cholesterol Education Panel (United States).

The EAS describes five phenotypic therapeutic groups based on plasma lipoprotein levels which are summarized in Table 19.5. Restriction of dietary saturated fats and cholesterol are suggested as the mainstay of therapy in group A and the initial therapeutic approach in group B patients. Group B patients may require medications with an LDL-C lowering effect to achieve the previously mentioned high and low risk therapeutic goals. Single-drug therapy suggested includes low doses of bile acid sequestrants, niacin, fibric acid derivatives or HMG CoA reductase inhibitors.

Group C patients, who are hypertriglyceridemics, should have underlying causes of hypertriglycerdemia eliminated. These include obesity, ethanol consumption, hydrochlorothiazide, beta blocker, and estrogen containing medications, and improved diabetes control when appropriate. Medications are generally not required, but suggested, are niacin or fibric acid derivatives.

The therapeutic recommendations for Group D are similar to those for Group B with the inclusion of suggested combined use of medications when necessary to affect cholesterol and triglyceride lowering. The setting of the group E patient where extreme elevations of plasma cholesterol and/or triglyceride are present the use of medications is usually inevitable to achieve the desired goals. This may require combination therapy, or consideration for referral to a specialized center.

Besides the lipid-lowering medications available by prescription in North America, the European market includes additional lipid lowering medications which are licensed for use in various countries. These include the following medications which are listed according to their chemical classification.

Fibric Acid Derivatives

- Beclofibrate
- Benzafibrate (Bezalip – MCP Pharmaceuticals Ltd., West Lothian, Scotland)
- Ciprofibrate
- Etofibrate
- Fenofibrate (Lipidil – Bristol-Myers Squibb and Lipanthyl – Fournier Ltd, Slough, UK)

These medications vary in dosage, and generally lower plasma VLDL and LDL (except in severe hypertriglyceridemia) levels and raise plasma HDL-C levels. Guidelines for the use of these medications is similar to that provided for gemfibrozil.

HMG CoA Reductase Inhibitors

- Pravastatin (Pravachol – Bristol-Myers Squibb)
- Simvastatin (Zocor – Merck)

These compounds can be provided at lower doses than lovastatin (Mevacor); pravastatin (Pravachol) 20 mg BID, and simvastatin (Zocor) 20 to 40 mg of which can be conveniently given as a single dosage. These medications have a powerful LDL-C lowering effect. Guidelines for the use of these medications are similar to those provided for lovastatin (Mevacor). Because the use of these medications has not been assessed in long term, prospective randomized placebo control trials, cautious use of these compounds is suggested until their therapeutic role is clearly defined.

TABLE 19.4 – **Conversion Factors**

Cholesterol	x	*Conversion Factor*		
mg/dl	x	0.02586	=	mmol/L
mmol/L	x	38.6698	=	mg/dl

Triglycerides	x	*Conversion Factor*		
mg/dl	x	0.01129	=	mmol/L
mmol/L	x	88.5740	=	mg/dl

TABLE 19.5 – **European Atherosclerosis Society Therapeutic Groupings Based on Plasma Lipid Levels**

Treatment Group	*Diagnostic Levels mg% (mmol/L)*
A	cholesterol 200-250 mg% (5.2-6.5 mmol/L) triglyceride <200 mg% (<2.3 mmol/L)
B	cholesterol 250-300 mg% (6.5-7.8 mmol/L) triglyceride <200 mg% (2.3 mmol/L)
C	cholesterol <200 mg% (5.2 mmol/L) triglyceride 200-300 mg% (2.3-5.6 mmol/L)
D	cholesterol 200-300 mg% (5.2-7.8 mmol/L) triglyceride 200-500 mg% (2.3-5.6 mmol/L)
E	cholesterol >300 mg% (>7.8 mmol/L) and/or triglyceride >500 mg% (>5.6 mmol/L)

References:

Buchwald H, Varro RL, Matts JP, et al: Effect of partial ileal bypass on mortality and morbidity from coronary heart disease in patients with hypercholesterolemia. Report from the Program on Surgical Control of the Hyperlipidemias (POSCH). N Engl J Med 1990;323:946.

The Expert Panel: Report of the National Cholesterol Education Program Expert Panel on detection, evaluation and treatment of high blood cholesterol in adults. Arch Intern Med 1988;148:36.

Gordon DJ, Probstfeld JL, et al: High density lipoprotein cholesterol and cardiovascular disease: four prospective American studies. Circulation 1989;79:8.

Grundy JM, Goodman DWS, et al.: The place of HDL in cholesterol management: a perspective of the National Cholesterol Education Program. Arch Intern Med 1989;149:505.

Lundberg GD, Iverson G, Radulescu G: Now read this: The SI units are here. JAMA 1986;255:2329.

Olson RE: A critique of the report of the National Institutes of Health Expert Panel on detection, evaluation and treatment of high blood cholesterol. Arch Intern Med 1989;149:1501.

Study Group, European Atherosclerosis Society: The recognition and management of hyperlipidemia in adults: A policy statement of the European Atherosclerosis Society. European Heart Journal 1988;9:571-600.

NOTES

#20 Dietary Fats and Plasma Lipids

Dietary Fats

The major dietary fats include cholesterol and triglyceride fats, the latter providing a source of dietary fatty acids. Fatty acids can be classified as saturated or unsaturated, depending on the absence or presence of double bonds in the carbon chain. Unsaturated fatty acids can be further subclassified as being either monounsaturated (one double bond) or polyunsaturated (more than one double bond).

Unsaturated fats can also be classified in terms of the position of the first double bond in the fatty acid chain by use of the omega system. According to this system, the terminal methyl group (the omega carbon of the fatty acid chain) is labeled the "omega" carbon.

Unsaturated fats containing the first double bond after the third carbon from the omega group are of the omega-3 series. Those possessing a first double bond after the sixth or ninth carbon from the omega carbon are omega-6 or omega-9 fatty acids, respectively. Table 20.1 lists commonly discussed dietary fats according to their classification and provides a list of dietary sources.

Recent studies have emphasized the importance of the position of the double bond in determining special biological effects of particular unsaturated fatty acids. In particular, marine oils (fish oils) of the omega-3 series have been implicated in lowering CAD risk (see Section #15). The omega-6 and omega-9 series are mainly found in terrestrial sources.

Oleic acid is an 18-carbon-long monounsaturated omega-9 series fatty acid, and linoleic polyunsaturated fatty acids belong to the omega-6 series. Although linolenic polyunsaturated fats belong to the omega-3 series, they come mainly from terrestrial sources and do not cause the biological effects of the marine omega-3 fatty acids (EPA and DHA). Although linoleic and linolenic acids are recognized as essential fatty acids because they cannot be synthesized by the body, their dietary requirements are small.

Dietary Fats and Cholesterol

The relationship of dietary fat intake to plasma cholesterol level is characterized by the Keys formula, developed from feeding studies involving dietary fats in humans. This formula is given in modified form for purposes of discussion below:

$$\text{plasma cholesterol level} = \sqrt{\text{dietary cholesterol}} + (2 \times \text{saturated fat intake} - \text{polyunsaturated fat intake})$$

Monounsaturated fats are not included in Keys' final equation because they did not appear to have a great effect on total plasma cholesterol levels. This equation emphasizes the basis for the current dietary recommendation provided in Section #19 and is further described in the following discussion.

Dietary Cholesterol

The recommended dietary cholesterol intake appears to be stringently low given the usual American diet, which is relatively high in cholesterol content. (One egg yolk contains approximately 250 mg.) This is because, as is shown by the square root in Keys' equation, a greater plasma cholesterol level reduction with comparable amounts of dietary cholesterol reduction occurs at relatively lower levels of dietary cholesterol intake.

This corresponds with cholesterol feeding studies which show that a ceiling for plasma cholesterol lowering exists between cholesterol intake and plasma cholesterol levels.

Until dietary cholesterol is reduced to 400 to 500 mg or less per day, plasma cholesterol levels will not be greatly affected. Thus, reducing dietary cholesterol will not greatly impact plasma cholesterol levels until it can be reduced to amounts below this ceiling. This is why current recommendations for cholesterol intake are very stringent.

The major sources of cholesterol are animal products, including:

- Meats (especially organ meats)
- Cheese
- Eggs

The previous identification of shrimp, oysters and lobsters as high-cholesterol foods is weakened with the recognition that some of the sterols are not cholesterol, but rather sea sterols. In addition, they have a lesser content of saturated fat and the presence of fatty acids of the omega-3 series. Recent finding indicate that oysters, clams, crab and mussels tend to lower plasma VLDL triglycerides and (except for mussels) LDL-C. Squid and shrimp are lipid neutral.

Saturated Fatty Acids

The direct relationship between dietary saturated fatty acid consumption and plasma cholesterol levels is well borne out by the Seven Countries study and is exemplified by the coefficient of two in the modified Keys' equation. Because of its powerful relationship to plasma cholesterol levels, current recommendations have been especially targeted on reducing dietary saturated fat intake.

Conversely, recent evidence indicates that stearic acid (18:0), a metabolic precursor of monounsaturated fatty acids, may have a neutral effect on plasma lipid levels compared with other saturated fats, in particular:

- Lauric acid (12:0)
- Myristic acid (14:0)
- Palmitic acid (16:0)

All of these saturated fatty acids are hypercholesterolemic.

A patient should be urged to eliminate the following major sources of dietary fats:

- Red meats
- Whole milk
- Cheese
- Hydrogenated fats
- Coconut oil

Polyunsaturated Fats

Polyunsaturated fat intake has been shown to have a cholesterol-lowering effect. This reflects the result of reductions in both plasma LDL-C and HDL-C lipoprotein fractions.

Because of the prominent effect on plasma LDL-C lowering, increased polyunsaturated fat intake has traditionally been viewed favorably for its lipid-modifying effects. This enthusiasm has been recently tempered by studies showing a direct association between increasing quantities of dietary polyunsaturated fat intake and increased incidence of certain forms of cancer.

In addition, there is no example of a free-living population that consumes a diet high in polyunsaturates. For this reason, current dietary recommendations do not promote polyunsaturated fat intake to the extent that has occurred in the past. However, Omega-3 fatty acids (fish oil) are a special class of polyunsaturated fats (see Section #15). The usual sources of polyunsaturated fats include margarines and other nonhydrogenated oils such as:

- Safflower
- Corn
- Soybean

Monounsaturated Fats

Findings that monounsaturated fat intake lowers plasma LDL-C levels without reducing plasma HDL-C levels has resulted in a resurgence of Mediterranean-style cooking. Recently, dietary enrichment with monounsaturates has been shown to reduce LDL susceptability to oxidative modification. In this style of cookery, olive oil, a large source of monounsaturated fat, is substituted for the saturated fats often used in the United States. In addition, monounsaturated fat intake has not borne any relationship to increased cancer risk.

Alternatively, these findings are challenged by recent studies showing no difference in plasma HDL-C levels in diets enriched in poly or mono-unsaturates.

Examples of human populations deriving large amounts of their dietary fat as monounsaturates exist, whereas no cultures typically consuming large amounts of polyunsaturated fats have been identified. Thus, dietary recommendations which favor monounsaturates seem appropriate.

Dietary recommendations of monounsaturated fat intake are now more liberal than in the past. The best dietary sources of monounsaturated fats include:

- Olive oil
- Canola oil (made from the rapeseed plant)
- Avocado oil

Atherogenic Index (Cholesterol-Saturated Fats)

Although plants do not make cholesterol and, therefore, do not provide a dietary source of cholesterol, plants can be a significant source of saturated fats. Saturated fats are widely used in the food industry because they have a long shelf life. They do not tend to go rancid, unlike polyunsaturated fats. Widely used for this purpose are:

- Coconut oil
- Palm oil
- Hydrogenated vegetable oil

CAVEAT: Although plant oils do not have cholesterol, those that have saturated oils pose an atherosclerotic risk in terms of their saturated fat content.

Table 20.2 lists foods according to their cholesterol-saturated fat index (CSI). A higher CSI indicates increasing atherogenicity. Note that processed foods can represent a typically overlooked source of saturated fat.

Dietary Fat and Regression

In a two year follow-up study in the dietary intervention only (placebo) group in the CLAS study increased risk of new lesions occured with both increased levels of total and polyunsaturated fat. The outcome of this trial supports the belief that restriction of saturated fat intake can reverse atherosclerosis, yet suggests that dietary saturated fat is best replaced by carbohydrate energy rather than mono- and polyunsaturates.

References

Blankenhorn DH, Johnson RL, Mack WJ, Elzein H, Vailas LI: The Influence of new lesions in human coronary arteries. JAMA 1990;263:1646.

Bonanome A, Grundy JM: Effect of dietary stearic acid on plasma cholesterol and lipoprotein levels. N Engl J Med 1988;318:1244.

Childs MT, Dorsett CS, King IB, Ostrander JC, Yamanaka WK: Effects of shellfish consumption on lipoproteins in normolipemia men. Am J Clin Nutr 1990;51:1020.

Connor SL, Gustafson JR, et al: The cholesterol/saturated fat index: an indication of the hyper-cholesterolemic and atherogenic potential of foods. Lancet 1986;1:1229.

Connor SL, Gustafson JR, et al: The cholesterol-saturated fat index for coronary prevention: background, use and a comprehensive table of foods. JAMA 1989;89:807.

Council on Scientific Affairs: Saturated fatty acids in vegetable oils. JAMA 1990;263:693.

Dreon DM, Vranizan KM, Krauss RM, Austin MA, Wood PD: The effects of polyunsaturated fat vs monounsaturated fat on plasma lipoproteins. JAMA 1990;263:2462.

Keys A, Anderson JT, Grande F: Prediction of serum cholesterol responses of man to changes of fats in the diet. Lancet 1957;1:948.

Glueck CJ, Connor WE: Diet-coronary heart disease relationship reconnoitered. Am J Clin Nutr 1985;31:727.

Goodnight SH, Harris WE, et al: Polyunsaturated fatty acids, hyperlipidemia and thrombosis. Arteriosclerosis 1982;2:87.

Grundy JM: Comparison of monounsaturated fats and carbohydrates for plasma cholesterol lowering. N Engl J Med 1986;314:745.

Grundy JM: Monounsaturated fatty acids, plasma cholesterol and coronary heart disease. Am J Clin Nutr 1987;45:1168.

Nestel PJ: Polyunsaturated fatty acids (n-3, n-6). Am J Clin Nutr 1987;45:1161.

Pyorala K: Dietary cholesterol in relation to plasma cholesterol and coronary heart disease. Am J Clin Nutr 1987;45:1176.

Reaven P, Parthasarathy S, Grosse BJ, et al: Feasibility of using an oleate-rich diet to reduce the susceptibility of low-density lipoprotein to oxidative modification in humans. Am J Clin Nutr 1991;54:701.

Rozenberg IH, Schaefer EJ: Dietary saturated fatty acids and blood cholesterol. N Engl J Med 1988;318:1270.

NOTES

TABLES 20.1 – 20.2 →

TABLE 20.1 — **Important Dietary Fatty Acids and Their Sources**

SATURATED FATTY ACIDS		
Nonhypercholesterolemic		
Stearic acid	18:0	Animal fats, certain vegetables
Hypercholesterolemic		
Palmitic acid	16:0	Tropical oils (palm, coconut, cocoa butter)
Myristic acid	14:0	
UNSATURATED FATTY ACIDS		
Mono		
Oleic acid	18:1 omega-9	Poultry, olive oil, canola oil, avocado, peanuts
Poly		
Linoleic acid	18:2 omega-6	Vegetable oils, specifically soybean, peanut and walnut oils
Linolenic acid	18:3 omega-3	
Arachidonic acid	20:4 omega-6	
Omega-3 Fatty Acids		
Eicosapentaenoic acid	20:5 omega-3	Marine oils
Docosahexaenoic acid	22:6 omega-3	

TABLE 20.2—**Cholesterol Saturated Fat Index of Selected Foods**

Food Item	CSI
White fish	4
Peanut butter	5
Poultry, no skin	6
Whole milk	7
Mayonnaise	10
Vegetable margarine	10
Ice cream	13
Beef, pork, lamb (20% fat)	13
Cheese (32 to 38% fat)	26
Eggs, whole (2)	29
Coconut oil, palm oil, cocoa butter	47

(Modified from Lancet 1986;1:1229, reprinted with permission.)

#21 Dietary Fiber

Dietary Fibers and Plasma Lipids

Although dietary fiber is typically thought of as roughage, it is a complex mixture of compounds classified according to water solubility. The classic roughage fibers are water-insoluble, structural fibers such as:

- Cellulose
- Lignin
- Certain hemicelluloses

Soluble fibers include the gel-forming substances such as:

- Pectins
- Gums
- Mucilages
- Remaining hemicelluloses

The soluble forms of fiber have been shown to reduce plasma cholesterol values. The major effect appears to be restricted to plasma LDL-C lowering. Although the mechanism of action is uncertain, it may be related to the ability of these fibers to bind bile acids in the intestinal lumen.

Fiber Recommendations

Although the exact amount of LDL-C lowering potentially caused by dietary soluble fiber consumption is not clear, the current evidence suggests that the effect is more prominent for individuals with higher plasma cholesterol levels. In general, a 10 percent reduction in plasma total and LDL-C can be anticipated by increasing dietary water-soluble fiber intake. Unfortunately, precise guidelines for exact amounts of dietary fiber are not available. Furthermore, they have been recently challenged by evidence that no difference occurred in plasma lipids and lipoproteins in normolipemic individuals between diets which contained either an isocaloric high-fiber oat bran or a low-fiber refined wheat supplement. However, the findings from this recent report may be consistent with previous studies because their baseline plasma cholesterol levels were low and may not have been anticipated to be greatly affected by the increased water soluble fiber intake during the oat bran phase.

A suggested increase in both soluble and insoluble dietary fibers above the customary Western diet is desirable. Rich sources of water-soluble fibers that should be emphasized include:

- Legumes (beans)
- Oat bran
- Corn
- Barley
- Sweet potatoes
- Yams
- Rice (gums)
- Apples
- Citrus fruits (pectin)

Recent studies indicate that daily ingestion of psyllium (three packets per day), commonly used as a bulk-forming stool agent, has comparable LDL-C lowering effects. Alternatively, formularies containing methylcellulose and calcium polycarbophil do not have this effect.

Fiber intake should be advanced gradually to avoid potential side effects. The typical gastrointestinal disturbances related to fiber consumption result from the products released from bacterial fiber fermentation and usually resolve within 24 to 48 hours as the intestine adapts to this uncustomary nutrient.

References

Anderson JW, Chen W-JL: Plant fiber: carbohydrate and lipid metabolism. Am J Clin Nutr 1979;32:346.

Anderson JW, Flore TL, Bazel Geil F, et al: Hypocholesterolemic effect of different bulk-forming hydrophilic fibers as adjuncts to dietary therapy in mild to moderate hypercholesterolemia. Arch Intern Med 1991;151:1597.

Anderson JW, Story L, et al: Hypocholesterolemic effects of oat bran or bean intake for hypercholesterolemic men. Am J Clin Nutr 1984;40:1146.

Connor WE: Dietary fiber, nostrum or critical nutrient? N Engl J Med 1990;322:193.

Council on Scientific Affairs. Dietary fiber and health. JAMA 1989;262:542.

Miettinen TA: Dietary fiber and lipids. Am J Clin Nutr 1987;45:1237.

Swain JF, Rouse IL, Curley CB, Sacks FM: Comparison of the effects of oat bran and low-fiber wheat on serum lipoprotein levels and blood pressure. N Engl J Med 1990;322:147.

#22 Ethanol

Ethanol Intake and CAD

The U-shaped relationship between the amount of reported ethanol (ETOH) intake and CAD risk has been established for both men and women. Compared with nondrinkers, CAD risk is reduced in moderate drinkers but increases curvilinearly with increased ethanol intake exceeding two drinks per day.

Varied sources of ethanol and their respective ethanol measurements are as follows:

- Beer (12 oz. or 350 ml) – 13.2 g
- Wine (4 oz. or 120 ml) – 10.8 g
- Liquor (one standard drink) – 15.1 g

The mechanism for the probable CAD risk protection from moderate ethanol intake is uncertain but could involve ethanol-induced increases in plasma HDL-C levels. It could also be related to psychological or blood pressure effects occurring with ethanol ingestion. The evidence for plasma HDL-C as a possible mechanism for mediating ethanol-induced CAD risk reduction, however, is controversial because the HDL-C_3 subfraction (unrelated to CAD risk) appears to be increased by ethanol consumption rather than HDL-C_2. In addition, recent findings indicate that drinking patterns influence plasma lipids. Weekend (binge) drinking raises LDL-C and apo-B in contrast. The same amount of ethanol ingestion spread out over a week lowers LDL-C and raises the HDL_2/HDL_3-C ratio.

Guidelines

Given the social and medical issues related to alcoholism and ethanol abuse, ethanol consumption should not be recommended, especially for nondrinkers. Ethanol as a source of calories is best eliminated from the diet for weight-loss purposes. In addition, ethanol intake increases plasma triglyceride levels and should be avoided by hypertriglyceridemic patients

References

Friedman LA, Kimball AW: Coronary heart disease mortality and alcohol consumption in Framingham. Am J Epidemiol 1986;124:481.

Hojnack TV, Deschenes RN, Clvette-Brown JE, et al: Effect of drinking pattern on plasma lipoproteins and body weight. Atherosclerosis 1991;88:49.

Moore RD, Pearson TA: Moderate alcohol consumption and coronary artery disease: a review. Medicine 1986;65:242.

Shaper AG, Wannamethee G, Walker M: Alcohol and mortality in British men: explaining the U-shaped curve. Lancet 1988;2:1267.

Stampfer MJ, Colditz GA, et al: A prospective study of moderate alcohol consumption and the risk of coronary disease and stroke in women. N Engl J Med 1988;319:267.

#23 Non-Dietary Measures

Smoking Cessation

Although the adverse relationship between CAD risk and cigarette smoking is well established, it should also be noted that cigarette smoking tends to lower plasma HDL-C levels. This aspect of smoking can be used as an additional incentive for smoking cessation, especially for a patient with depressed plasma HDL-C levels.

Physical Activity and Exercise

Increased levels of leisure-time physical activity maintained throughout adulthood are associated with decreased CAD risk. Although physical activity does not necessarily equate with exercise training per se, exercise training has been shown to raise plasma HDL-C levels and reduce plasma triglyceride levels.

An exercise intervention study in a group of men indicates that achieving a threshold of approximately eight miles (12.9 km) a week through jogging is necessary to raise plasma HDL-C levels by 10 percent after a one year period. This mileage represents approximately 1,200 k/cal of energy expenditure per week.

Recently the recognized effect of exercise training on reducing plasma triglyceride levels and raising plasma HDL-C levels (HDL_2-C subfraction) has been shown to occur independently of concomitant reductions in body fat. Regular participation in physical activity pursuits should be recommended for all individuals, not only for weight management issues but also to improve cardiovascular fitness and reduce CAD risk.

Physical exercise is currently one of the few available nonpharmacologic methods, along with weight reduction and cigarette smoking cessation, for raising plasma HDL_2-C levels.

References

Crique MH, Cowan LD, et al: Lipoproteins as mediators for the effect of alcohol consumption and cigarette smoking on cardiovascular mortality: results from the Lipid Research Clinics follow-up study. Am J Epidemiol 1987;126:629.

Paffenbarger RS, Wing AL, Hyde RT: Physical activity as an index of heart attack risk in college alumni. Am J Epidemiol 1978;108:161.

Powell KE, Thompson PD, et al: Physical activity and the incidence of coronary heart disease. Ann Rev Public Health 1987;8:253.

Stubbe I, Eskilsson J, Nilsson-Ehle P: High-density lipoprotein concentrations increase after stopping smoking. Br Med J 1982;284:1511.

Wood PD, Haskell WL, et al.: Increased exercise level and plasma lipoprotein concentration: a one-year, randomized, controlled study in sedentary, middle-aged men. Metabolism 1983;32:31.

Wood PD, Stefanick ML, et al: Changes in plasma lipids and lipoproteins in overweight men during weight loss through dieting as compared with exercise. N Engl J Med 1989;319:1173.

#24 Dietary Therapy: Outcome and Goals

Anticipated Outcome of Non-Dietary Interventions

The patient who has adhered to the current dietary recommendation can expect a 10 to 20 percent reduction in plasma cholesterol levels. Greater reductions have occurred for some.

It should be noted that in certain groups, particularly during pregnancy, this advice should be liberalized in view of the need for increased dietary iron intake.

In contrast, individuals with certain genetically determined dyslipidemias, particularly that of familial hypercholesterolemia, can be relatively resistant to plasma cholesterol lowering by dietary measures alone. These patients can be more quickly initiated to medication therapy after several months of dietary intervention alone.

Therapeutic Goals (For Dietary Intervention)

The desired results for dietary intervention are to attain plasma LDL-C levels that are less than:

- 130 mg% (3.4 mmol/L) in high risk patients*
- 160 mg% (4.1 mmol/L) in non-high risk patients

***Note:** The findings from recent regression studies support LDL-C lowering below 100 mg% (2.6 mmol/L) in patients with established CAD discussed in Section #1.

NOTES

24.

#25 Children

Pathogenic Evidence

The study of CAD in younger populations is hampered by the inability to provide direct evidence of cause and effect between CAD risk factors and CAD events in children. In addition, it is controversial whether the fatty streaks ubiquitously found in the artery intimal layers during early life truly represent morphological findings of precursor lesions to the atherosclerotic plaque lesions characteristic of advanced CAD.

Atherosclerosis should not be viewed as a purely adult phenomenon. Autopsy studies from healthy soldiers killed in combat in both the Korean and Vietnam wars provide evidence of atherosclerotic plaque formation in these asymptomatic young adults.

Autopsy evidence from the Bogalusa Heart Study indicates that the extent of atherosclerosis in children is related to their CAD risk-factor status. Autopsy data from 35 individuals (including eight cigarette smokers) of ages ranging from five to 24 years indicated that antemortem plasma VLDL-C and LDL-C levels were directly correlated and plasma HDL-C levels were inversely correlated to the extent of coronary artery lesions independent of age, race and gender. These findings have been corroborated by the Pathobiological Determinants of Atherosclerosis in Youth (PDAY) Research Group in 390 males of ages 15 to 34 years.

The strong association between plasma LDL-C levels and extent of aortic fatty streaks in both black and white children has been confirmed. Similarly, serum cholesterol levels have been directly correlated with increasing levels of atherosclerotic indices based on autopsy studies in 2,856 subjects of ages three months to 30 years involved in a Japanese nationwide study.

Familial hypercholesterolemia also served as evidence that severely elevated plasma LDL-C levels, which are especially pronounced in the homozygotic form of this disorder, are associated with advanced stages of atherosclerosis at an early age.

Certainly inheritance is an important determinant of both plasma cholesterol levels and CAD risk. Male relatives of children classified into high plasma cholesterol strata were shown to have a twofold excess of CAD mortality compared with children with lower plasma cholesterol levels. These findings, and evidence from other studies, support the importance of identifying hypercholesterolemic children for early intervention. Interestingly, elevated Lp(a) levels are found in white, but not black, children who have a high prevalence of parenteral myocardial infarction. A study in the Netherlands found the sons of fathers with severe CAD to have higher levels of apo-B and the apo-B/apo-A-I ratio than sons of fathers free of atherosclerosis.

Because relative CAD risk-factor rankings within groups of children tend to persist into adulthood (tracking) according to some but not all studies, and to increase in severity during maturation, CAD risk-factor intervention is an important aspect of primary prevention.

Plasma Lipids During Childhood

Dramatic changes in plasma levels of lipids and lipoproteins occur during the first year of life, when mean levels of plasma cholesterol markedly rise to near adult levels by one to two years of age. Plasma levels of lipids and lipoproteins are related more to the physiological development of sexual maturation than to chronologic age alone.

Gender differences in plasma HDL-C levels occur at puberty, at which time a decline in this lipoprotein value occurs in boys but not in girls. This gender difference persists into adulthood and is purported to account for relative risk differences for CAD between men and women. Levels of apolipoproteins appear to mirror those of their respective lipoprotein particles.

Cholesterol Screening in Children

Not only does the extent of CAD risk factors in children predict risk-factor severity in their parents, but also the converse is true. The Princeton School Family Study found that twice as many offspring of hypercholesterolemics have elevated levels of total cholesterol and LDL-C than the offspring of normocholesterolemic parents. However, the use of family history as a predictive screen for hypercholesterolemia has not been shown to be useful, possibly because at the young childhood age the parents history of CAD is an insensitive predictor because it is still an indeterminant. Alternatively, recent findings from the Muscaline Study show that general cholesterol screening when repeated on several occasions during childhood greatly over-estimated those requiring treatment based on their adult values. Findings from the Bogalusa Heart Study show good tracking from childhood to young adulthood. Because of the poor long term predictive value of low cholesterol levels (according to some studies), it has been argued that for most individuals cholesterol screening could cause a disservice to them by giving them a false since of security.

Although the widespread routine practice of cholesterol screening among adolescents is controversial, it has been argued that children in a high-risk setting should be screened based on family history. Also, it has been argued because of the strong tracking phenomenon of plasma cholesterol levels during maturation, a one-time screening assessment to identify those at high risk for future reassessment is a reasonable public health approach. However, the most recent sentiment based on the previous discussion appears to be that the benefits do not outweigh the risks. Routine screening of lipids is not recommended for infants.

In the setting of familial hypercholesterolemia, cord blood should be sent for a determination of plasma cholesterol level because this diagnosis can be made at birth (and even before with amniocentesis) and early institution of therapy can be appropriated. Hypertriglyceridemia screening is not useful except in the high-risk patient at 10 years of age.

Treatment – Public Health Measures and General Guidelines

Although initiation of public health measures to lower plasma cholesterol levels in infancy is controversial, infants fed a low-cholesterol, low-saturated fat diet had lower plasma cholesterol levels at six months and three years of age than did control subjects. Educational programs provided at the grade school level appear to reduce dietary saturated fat intake and plasma cholesterol levels favorably.

A prudent diet similar to the Step 1 recommendations for adults is probably appropriate dietary advice for children over two years of age. This is especially relevant in view of the concerns of childhood-onset obesity believed to stem from the growing level of physical inactivity and increased consumption of dietary fat by this nation's youth, as shown in Table 25.1.

Because of the concern that a diet restricted in dietary fat may prevent optimal myelinization and development of the central nervous system, it is suggested that dietary fat restriction not be employed until after two years of age. Breast milk contains 40 to 50 percent calories as fat and 150 mg/dl cholesterol. It should be considered as the gold standard of diet for the first year.

Other hygienic health habits that can be suitably altered and maintained by involving parental support include smoking cessation and participation in physical activity. It is currently suggested that a target level of total plasma cholesterol be below 170 mg% (4.4 mmol/L) (plasma LDL-C level below 110 mg% [1.7 mmol/L]).

Pediatric Primary Lipid Disorders and Therapy

Familial Hypercholesterolemia

This disorder can be diagnosed from the cord blood of offspring with an appropriate family history for this condition. Dietary restriction of saturated fat (less than seven percent of daily caloric intake and cholesterol – less than 200 mg/day) is required, and the use of bile acid sequestrants can be used with attention given to fat-soluble vitamin intake (vitamins A and D).

Current long-term therapy data using other agents is not available on a controlled study basis, although the use of HMG-CoA reductase inhibitors may be considered in the homozygote.

More aggressive forms of therapy, including liver transplantation (to provide a source of LDL receptors) and plasma LDL apheresis (to lower the plasma levels of the putative LDL-C lipoprotein) may also be necessary in the homozygote. However, it is prudent to consult with a specialist in this setting.

Other Hypercholesterolemias

Primary dyslipidemias seen in adulthood can exist in childhood. In particular, children who are identifed as hypercholesterolemic should be given dietary intervention, although the use of medications is best withheld (except in severe forms) until adulthood, because little is known regarding the long-term effects of pharmaceutical agents in adolescence.

Familial Hyperchylomicronemia

This very rare autosomal recessive disorder exists with isolated fasting chylomicronemia (Frederickson-Levy Type I). This results from the congenital absence of lipoprotein lipase LPL or deficiency of apo-CII, which activates this enzyme's activity. The presence of LPL activity can be detected after heparin injection, which activates LPL and should normally cause chylomicronemia to decline with the concomitant production of plasma free fatty acids.

These findings will not occur in the setting of this disorder. Two-thirds of those with this disorder are usually seen before age 10 for abdominal pain which may be due to pancreatitis or enlargement of the viscera because of their distension with lipids. Eruptive xanthomas and lipemia retinalis can also be noted. Premature CAD is not a recognized complication of this disorder, possibly because the lack of chylomicron metabolism prevents the formation of atherogenic remnant lipoprotein particles.

No pharmaceutical therapy is available for this rare condition, which can be treated with total fat restriction to less than 0.5 g/kg/day (or less than 10 percent calories of fat per day). Medium-chain triglycerides can be given as a food supplement to provide dietary calories, as they do not require chylomicron formation for absorption.

Other Hypertriglyceridemias

Hypertriglyceridemia does not typically appear during childhood; therefore, screening is useless except in high-risk patients age 10 and older.

References

Barness LA: Cholesterol in children. JAMA 1986;256:2871.

Berensen GS, Blonde CV, et al: Cardiovascular risk factor variables during the first year of life. Am J Dis Children 1979;133:1049.

Committee on Nutrition, American Academy of Pediatrics: Prudent life-style for children: dietary fat and cholesterol. Pediatrics 1986;78:521.

Coughenour MC: Functional aspects of food consumption activity and family life cycle stages. J Marriage Family 1972;34:656.

Enos WF, Beyer JC, Holmes RH: Pathogenesis of coronary disease in American soldiers killed in Korea. JAMA 1955;148:912.

Freedman DS, et al: Black-white differences in aortic fatty streaks in adolescence and early adulthood: the Bogalusa Heart Study. Circulation 1988;77:856.

Friedman G, Goldberg SJ: An evaluation of the safety of the low-saturated fat, low-cholesterol diet, beginning in infancy. Pediatrics 1985;58:655.

Garcia RE, Moodie DS: Routine cholesterol surveillance in childhood. Pediatrics 1989;84:751.

Glueck CJ: Pediatric primary prevention of atherosclerosis. N Engl J Med 1986;314:175.

Glueck CJ, et al: Hypercholesterolemia and hypertriglyceridemia in children: a pediatric approach to primary atherosclerosis prevention. Am J Dis Children 1974;128:569.

Griffin TC, Christoffel KK, Birrs HJ, et al: Family history evaluation as a preventive screen for childhood hypercholesterolemia. Pediatrics 1989;84:365.

Holtzman NA: The great cholesterol. Pediatrics 1991;87:943.

Killen JD, et al: Cardiovascular disease risk reduction in tenth graders, a multiple-factor, school-based approach. JAMA 1988;260:1728.

Lauer RM, Clarke WR: Use of cholesterol measurements in childhood for the prediction of adult hypercholesterolemia. The Muscatine Study. JAMA 1990;264:3034.

Lew EA: Some implications of mortality statistics relating to coronary artery disease. J Chron Dis 1957;6:192.

McNamara JJ, et al: Coronary artery disease in combat casualties in Vietnam. JAMA 1971; 216:1185.

Morrison JA, et al: Familial associations of lipids and lipoproteins in families of hypercholesterolemic probands. Arteriosclerosis 1982;2:151.

Newman TB, Browner WS, Hulley SB: The case against childhood cholesterol screening. JAMA 1990;264:3039.

PDAY Research Group: Relationship of atherosclerosis in young men to serum lipoprotein cholesterol concentration and smoking. JAMA 1990;264:3018.

Position statement: Diagnosis and treatment of primary hyperlipidemia in childhood. Circulation 1986;74:1181A.

Puska P, et al: The North Karelia Youth Project: Estimation of two years of intervention on health behavior and CVD risk factors among 13- to 15-year-old children. Prevent Med 1982;11:550.

Roberts WC: Fast foods and quick placques. Am J Cardiol 1987;59:721.

Srinivasan SR, Dahlen GH, Jarpa RA, et al: Racial (black-white) differences in serum lipoprotein (a) distribution and its relation to parental myocardial infarction in children. Bogalusa Heart Study. Circulation 1991;84:160.

Summary of recommendations of the Conference on Blood Lipids in Children: Optimal levels for early prevention of coronary artery disease. Prevent Med 1983;12:728.

Tanaka K, et al: A nationwide study of atherosclerosis in infants, children and young adults in Japan. Atherosclerosis 1988;72:143.

Tell GS, et al: Cholesterol, high-density lipoprotein cholesterol and triglycerides during puberty: the Oslo Youth Study. Am J Epidemiol 1985; 122:750.

Van Stiphout WAHJ, Hofman A, Kruijssen HACM, et al: Is the ratio of ApoB/ApoA-I an early prediction of coronary atherosclerosis? Atherosclerosis 1986;62:179.

Welter HJ, et al: Modification of risk factors for coronary heart disease. Five-year results of a school-based intervention trial. N Engl J Med 1988;318:1039.

Webber LS, Srinivajan SR, Wattigney WA, et al: Tracking of serum lipids and lipoproteins from childhood to adulthood. Bogalusa Heart Study. Am J Epi 1991;133:884.

TABLE 25.1 – **Fast Food Composition**

Company/Product	Calories	Fat (tsp)	Sodium (mg)
	Quantity in a Typical Serving		
Burgers			
Wendy's Kid's Meal Hamburger	200	2	210
McDonald's Hamburger	263	3	506
Hardee's Big Deluxe	503	7	903
Burger King Whopper	626	9	482
Jack-in-the-Box Jumbo Jack (with cheese)	630	8	1,665
Wendy's Triple Cheeseburger	1,040	15	1,848
Fries			
Arby's French Fries	211	2	30
Arthur Treacher's Chips	276	3	39
Burger King French Fries (regular)	227	3	160
Hardee's French Fries (large)	406	5	306
Shakes			
Jack-in-the-Box Strawberry	320	2	240
Burger King Vanilla (10 fl. oz.)	321	2	205
Hardee's Milk Shake (11 fl. oz.)	391	2	241
Burger King Chocolate (10 fl. oz.)	374	3	225
Dairy Queen Chocolate (large: 21 fl. oz.)	990	6	360

(Modified from Roberts WC, Fast foods and quick plaques. Am J Cardiol 59:721-723;1987. Reprinted with permission.)

#26 The Elderly

CAD in the Elderly

Although age 65 is generally used as a demarcation of old age, this is not based on a specific physiological correlate. It is a historical definition created by General Otto von Bismarck as a means of forcing recalcitrant generals into retirement.

Despite the absence of specific criteria to define "elderly," it is well recognized that the segment of older Americans is growing at a pace far surpassing other age groups. Individuals achieving 65 years of age can be expected to live an additional 17 years. The group of Americans aged 65 and older accounts for nearly 30 percent of the nation's health care costs. Because CAD represents a major disease problem (accounting for more than 70 percent of all mortality in those 75 years of age and older), reduction of CAD in this population group will become an increasing priority with our graying society.

CAD Risk Factors in the Elderly

Although CAD risk factors are well recognized in middle-aged populations, controversy exists regarding the relationship of some of these factors to CAD risk, particularly plasma cholesterol levels in older age groups. The Framingham Study shows a general decline in plasma LDL-C levels in men, whereas, a mild increase occurs in women after the age of 65 years.

Although postmenopausal women experience a decline in plasma HDL-C levels, the higher plasma

HDL-C levels in women persist into old age. In contrast, menopause is associated with a rise in plasma LDL-C levels, which increase to the female's levels above their male counterpart's, a trend that continues into old age.

For women, a continued increase in plasma total cholesterol/HDL-C ratio occurs after menopause and continues into old age, which may explain the relative increased postmenopausal CAD risk.

For men, this ratio plateaus at approximately age 55 but remains higher than that in women. The incidence of hypercholesterolemia declines for both men and women with old age. The rate of incidence in men aged 65 to 74 averages 16.6 percent and drops to 9.4 percent at ages 85 to 94. In the women's category, the percentage of 39.7 in those aged 65 to 74 drops to 18.4 in the 85 to 94 age bracket.

Plasma total cholesterol levels are not as closely related to CAD risk in elderly populations as in their younger counterparts, although recent findings from the Honolulu Heart Program indicate that total plasma cholesterol levels do persist as an independent predictor of CAD risk in men over 65 years of age. In addition to an apparently stronger association with increased CAD risk with total plasma cholesterol levels in women, plasma triglyceride values also appear to bear an independent CAD risk relationship in older women. Recent findings from the Framingham Study indicate that plasma HDL-C levels are the most predictive lipid parameter with respect to CAD risk. 26.

Although plasma HDL-C levels appear to represent the most important CAD risk predictor in the elderly and because current CAD risk screening recommendations include total plasma cholesterol and not plasma HDL-C, the selective measurement of plasma HDL-C levels in those with identified hypercholesterolemia ignores the group of CAD risk elderly with low plasma total-C and HDL-C.

Recommendations

Especially in view of the fact that a 65-year-old will likely live another 20 years, dyslipidemia as a CAD risk factor should not be ignored in the elderly because of its potential bearing on this important chronic disease. In addition, because the presence of hypercholesterolemia is more prevalent in the elderly than in other age groups, this represents a higher risk population. Unfortunately, there is a lack of intervention trials in CAD risk-factor reduction and CAD outcome in the elderly, although at present such a study is underway.

Based on the findings in other age groups and on recent evidence supporting the relationship between LDL-C reduction and regression of atherosclerosis, efforts aimed at the management of lipid disorders are important in the elderly, especially for those individuals with CAD. Attention should also be given to other CAD risk factors which may coexist. Elderly women represent a particularly important group who are at male equivalent levels of CAD risk. Hypertriglyceridemia, especially in the presence of depressed plasma HDL-C levels and diabetes, warrants therapeutic consideration.

Although the dietary interventions using current Step 1 recommendations are appropriate in the elderly, the use of lipid-lowering agents presents a concern for increases in age-related side effects. Constipation often limits the effective use of bile acid sequestrants. In this setting, the use of three to four packets of psyllium per day may be an alternative.

The elderly may have a higher risk for the potential side effects caused by other pharmaceutic agents, in particular hepatic disorders. In view of the high prevalence of the use of multiple medications by older adults, issues regarding drug interactions are an important consideration in this group.

When using lipid-altering medications in the elderly, the clinician should be aware of potential side effects and be especially cautious in the use of these medications, perhaps emphasizing lower dosage regimens.

References

Abbott RD, et al: High-density cholesterol, total cholesterol screening and myocardial infarction: the Framingham Study. Arteriosclerosis 1988; 8:207.

Benfante R, Reed D: Is elevated cholesterol level a risk factor for coronary heart disease in the elderly? JAMA 1990;263:393.

Castelli WB, et al: The incidence of coronary artery disease in lipoprotein cholesterol levels: the Framingham Study. JAMA 1986;256:2835.

Denke MA, Grundy SM; Hypercholesterolemia in elderly persons: resolving the treatment dilemma. Ann Intern Med 1990;112:780.

Harris T, et al: Proportional hazards analysis of risk factors of coronary heart disease in individuals aged 65 or older: The Framingham Heart Study. J Am Geriat Soc 1988;36:1023.

Kafunek SD, Kwiterovick PD: Treatment of hypercholesterolemia in the elderly. Ann Intern Med 1990;112:780.

Kannel WB: Nutrition and the occurrence and prevention of cardiovascular disease in the elderly. Nutri Rev 1988;42:68.

Leon AS: Age and other predictors of coronary heart disease. Med Sci Sports Exercise 1987; 19:159.

Schaefer EJ, et al: Plasma lipoprotein in healthy octogenarians: lack of reduced high-density lipoprotein cholesterol levels, results from the Framingham Study. Metabolism 1989;38:293.

Zimetbaum P, Frishman W, Aronson M: Lipids, vascular disease and dementia with advancing age. Epidemiologic considerations. Arch Intern Med 1991;151:240.

#27 Women

CAD Risk in Women

Although women are considered to be protected from CAD relative to men, they are not immune. CAD is the leading cause of death in women, with nearly 250,000 women dying from atherosclerotic-related events yearly in the United States. The gender difference in CAD incidence has been attributed to various psychological and physiological differences, in particular gynecoid hormones, which appear to promote female protection. Current evidence indicates that estrogen confers female protection by promoting relative increases in plasma HDL-C levels. In addition, estrogen lowers plasma LDL-C by upregulating hepatic LDL receptor activity.

Population studies indicate a sex-related divergence in plasma HDL-C levels during childhood, with a greater decline in plasma HDL-C levels occurring in boys. During adulthood, women maintain higher plasma HDL-C levels (mean 55 mg% [1.4 mmol/L]) compared with their male counterparts (45 mg% [1.2 mmol/L]). This difference persists until menopause, when plasma estrogen influences decrease. At this time, women experience an increased:

- Ratio in plasma LDL-C/HDL-C
- Incidence in CAD events approaching those of men

In addition to the biological role of estrogen in raising plasma HDL-C levels, pharmacological use of estrogens raises plasma HDL-C levels.

Female Risk Factors

The following CAD risk factors are important considerations for both genders:

- Lipid disorders
- Cigarette smoking
- Hypertension
- Obesity (body fat distribution)
- Physical inactivity
- Psychosocial issues
- Family history of CAD

CAD risk factors which are of special importance for women are:

- Personal history of CAD
- Oral contraceptive use
- Postmenopausal estrogens
- Diabetes mellitus
- Lipids and lipoproteins

Personal History of CAD

Men and women have the same prognosis after suffering a myocardial infarction. The prognosis for coronary artery bypass grafting and angioplastic patients is worse for women than it is for men.

Oral Contraceptive Use

Evidence from the Nurse's Health Study suggests that the increased CAD risk associated with oral contraceptive use does not persist after oral contraceptive use is discontinued. It is further suggested that CAD events related to oral contraceptive use reported in earlier studies largely represent the results of prothrombogenic influences of estrogenic potency. In addition, progestinal agents have a tendency to lower plasma HDL-C levels. Current oral contraceptive formulas are lower-dose in both estrogenic (less thrombogenic) and progestinal effects, resulting in a balanced or plasma HDL-C-neutral effect. A paradoxical note in view of the increasing prevalence of cigarette smoking among young women is the documented synergistic increased CAD risk of cigarette smoking and oral contraceptive use.

Postmenopausal Estrogens

The postmenopausal use of conjugated and esterified estrogens is associated with:

- Increased levels of plasma HDL-C
- Decreased CAD risk

Although the use of combined estrogen-progestinal regimens with respect to CAD risk in the postmenopausal woman remains to be clearly defined (due to the plasma HDL-C-lowering effects of progestin), current evidence supports the role of postmenopausal estrogen in reducing CAD risk. This effect may be most pronounced in women with depressed levels of plasma HDL-C. A recent report indicates that the administration of postmenopausal estrogens prevents the anticipated decline of plasma HDL-C levels and the rise of plasma LDL-C levels, although plasma triglyceride levels increase above premenopausal levels. Precautions should be taken regarding the use of postmenopausal estrogens in hypertriglyceridemic women with the concern of exacerbating this condition. The effects of tamoxifen, which is a commonly used agent in the treatment of breast cancer, on plasma lipids mirrors those of estrogen, but has a lesser effect on HDL-C raising.

Diabetes Mellitus

This is a particularly important risk factor for women over 45 years of age. Diabetes mellitus has been shown to represent an independent CAD risk factor with a two-fold increased CAD risk. However, there appears to be a two-fold differential CAD risk between the genders, with women diabetics experiencing twice the CAD risk increase relative to males.

Lipids and Lipoproteins

Evidence suggests that hypertriglyceridemia may represent a particular CAD risk factor for women. In contrast to the negative findings for men, the Framingham Study has provided evidence that hypertriglyceridemia represents a CAD risk factor in older women independent of conventional CAD risk factors, including plasma HDL-C.

Overview

CAD currently is and may continue to grow as a major disease concern to women. Current understanding of CAD risk in women is limited by a lack of female-specific research in this area when compared to the usual research subject, the high-risk male.

The profile of the high-risk female includes the following gender-specific elements:

- Personal history of CAD/postmenopausal
- Diabetes mellitus
- Android body habitus (reflecting the presence of upper body/abdominal obesity)
- Family history of CAD
- Hypertriglyceridemia
- Depressed plasma HDL-C level

All aspects of patient management should be given particular attention to improve the CAD risk status of a women exhibiting these risk factors. Lipidologically, the best targets are efforts to raise plasma HDL-C levels and lower plasma triglycerides. These include:

- Weight reduction (when necessary)
- Increased physical activity
- Dietary adherence
- Use of appropriate medications aimed at plasma HDL-C raising when this is indicated (including estrogens)

Findings from a recent prospective randomized controlled study using combined medications to lower cholesterol in men and women with Familial Hypercholesterolemia showed evidence of regression occurred in the treatment group which correlated with reduced LDL-C in both women and men examined separately.

References

Barrett-Connor EL, Cohn BA, Wingard DL, et al: Why is diabetes mellitus a stronger risk factor for fatal ischemic heart disease in women than men? JAMA 1991;265:627.

Barrett-Connor E, Wingard DL: Sex differential in ischemic heart disease mortality in diabetics: a prospective population-based study. Am J Epidemiol 1983;118:489.

Bush TL, Barrett-Connor E, Cowan LD, et al: Cardiovascular mortality and noncontraceptive use of estrogen in women: results from the Lipid Research Clinics program follow-up study. Circulation 1987;75:1102.

Bush TL, Fried LP, Barrett-Connor E: Cholesterol, lipoproteins and coronary heart disease in women. Clin Chem 1988;34:B60.

Castelli WP: The triglyceride issue; a view from Framingham. Am Heart J 1986;112:432.

Cowley MJ, Mullin JM, et al: Sex differences in the results with coronary angioplasty. NHLBI PT(A). Circulation 1983;68(Suppl III):III-97.

Fiebach NH, Viscoli CM, Horwitz RI: Differences between women and men in survival after myocardial infarction: biology or methodology. JAMA 1990;263:1092.

Gordon T, Castelli WP, Hjortland MC, et al: High density lipoproteins and risk of coronary heart disease: The Framingham study. Am J Med 1977;62:707.

Greenland P, Reicher-Reiss H, Goldbourt U, et al: In-hospital and one year mortality in 1,524 women after myocardial infarction. Circulation 1991;83:484.

Hazzard WR: Atherogenesis: why women live longer than men. Geriatrics 1985;40:42.

Holden C: Why do women live longer than men? Science 1987;238:158.

Kane JP, Malloy MJ, Ports TA, et al: Regression of coronary atherosclerosis during treatment of Familial Hypercholesterolemia with combined drug regimens. JAMA 1990;264:3007.

Kannel WB, McGee DL: Diabetes and cardiovascular disease: The Framingham study. JAMA 1979;241:2035.

Knopp RH: Cardiovascular effects of endogenous and exogenous sex hormones over a woman's lifetime. Am J Obst Gynecol 1988;158:1630.

Leaf DA: A woman's heart. An update on coronary artery disease in women. West J Med 1988; 149:751.

Loop FD, Golding LR, MacMillan JP, et al: Coronary artery bypass surgery in women compared with men: analysis of risks and long-term results. J Am Coll Cardiol 1983;1:383.

Love RR, Wiebe DA, Newcomb PA, et al: Effects of tamoxifen on cardiovascular risk factors in postmenopausal women. Ann Intern Med 1991;115:860.

Mann JI, Vessey MP, Thorogood M, et al: Myocardial infarction in young women with special reference to oral contraceptive practice. Br M J 1975;2:241.

Matthews KA, Meilahn E, et al: Menopause and risk factors for coronary heart disease. N Engl J Med 1989;321:641.

Miscell DR: Contraception. N Engl J Med 1989; 320:777.

Rifkind BM, Segal P: Lipid research clinics reference values for hyperlipidemia and hypolipidemia. JAMA 1983;250:1969.

Smoking and Health: A national status report: a report to Congress. Publication No. HHJ/PHS/ CDC 87-8396. Rockville, MD: US DHHS, 1987.

Wahl P, Walden C, Knopp R, et al: Effect of estrogen/progestin potency on lipid/lipoprotein cholesterol. N Engl J Med 1983;308:862.

Walsh BW, Schiff I, Rosner B, et al: Effect of postmenopausal estrogen replacement on the concentration and metabolism of plasma lipoproteins. N Engl J Med 1991;325:1196.

Wenger NK: Coronary disease in women. Ann Rev Med 1985;36:285.

#28 Apolipoproteins and CAD Risk

Apolipoproteins and Lipoprotein Lp(a) and CAD Risk: An Overview

A growing body of research continues to support the important role of plasma apolipoproteins in CAD risk. Table 4.1 (see Section #4) summarized the currently recognized functions of some apolipoproteins. The relationship of apolipoproteins to CAD risk mirrors that of their associated lipoprotein; plasma apo-B (LDL-C) is positively and plasma apo-A (HDL-C) is inversely associated with CAD risk. These relationships are highly complex. Historically, lipoprotein metabolism and CAD risk have been characterized more extensively than has the more recently expanding field of apolipoprotein research. Indeed, apolipoprotein metabolism has provided important insights into CAD risk. However, the findings from a recent prospective study suggest that little predictive value of apo's -A-I, A-II, and B are apparent for CAD risk after other conventional risk factors are considered. Recently, Kottke et al, have provided normative standards of plasma apolipoprotein values in the Rochester Family Heart Study.

Hyperapobetalipoproteinemia is a disorder characterized by increased plasma apo-B levels in the setting of normocholesterolemia. This lipid disorder may explain why particular individuals suffer from CAD although their total plasma cholesterol levels are normal. Similarly, familial combined hyperlipidemia, which is associated with increased CAD risk, metabolically results from an overproduction of apo-B.

Although apolipoprotein studies will continue to show insightful perspectives in CAD research, it is not clear whether this will ultimately translate into the level of clinical applications that has been currently achieved by comparison with plasma lipoproteins, for the following reasons:

- Current public health issues requiring decades of effort to involve public and professional support demand a major refocusing of priorities
- Nationally standardized techniques for apolipoprotein measurement are not available; nor are normative population data
- Major clinical trials involving apolipoprotein modification and CAD risk outcome remain to be conducted

Although apolipoprotein levels do not currently conform to policy standards, an understanding of apolipoproteins and CAD risk is crucial for the practitioner who may seek further subspecialty referral for patient management and who must keep abreast of current medical knowledge. Awareness of apolipoprotein metabolism will continue to be in the forefront of the expansion of understanding CAD pathogenesis and therapy. Apolipoproteins will likely be included in the future as CAD risk factors. The issue of lipoprotein Lp(a) and CAD risk provides a similar discussion.

Apo-B System

Apo-B-100, the primary apolipoprotein of the LDL-C particle, has achieved a recognized indirect relationship with increased CAD risk. In addition, abnormal apolipoprotein B metabolism is demonstrated in two specific lipid disorders. An abnormality causing increased plasma apolipoprotein B levels relative to plasma LDL-C (i.e., an abnormally increased number of LDL particles versus a normal number of LDL particles having a high cholesterol content) has a suspected atherogenic role in hyperapobetalipoproteinemia. An increased influx of apo-B lipoproteins into the plasma is evident in familial combined hyperlipidemia. Currently, further work in developing standardized measurements of apo-B in addition to large-scale prospective intervention trials will be necessary to judge the clinical role of apo-B.

Apo-A System

Apo-A-I, which has a role in LCAT activation, appears to be the specific apolipoprotein of the apo-A series bearing a relationship to CAD risk. Associated with HDL-C, apo-A-I has a similar inverse relationship to CAD risk. As was discussed in Section #4, evidence indicates that HDL which contains only apo A-I (LpA-I) appears to be inversely related with CAD risk, while HDL containing both apo A-I and A-II (LpA-I: A-II) is inert in this respect. Like apo-B-100, further prospective clinical trials, as well as standardization in measurement, are required to make this a clinically useful measurement.

Apo-E System

Apo-E abnormalities are associated with atherogenic dyslipidemia, also known as familial dysbetalipoproteinemia (Type III or broad band disease). This occurs due to the partial or complete absence of apo-E or an abnormal isoform of apo-E. In fact, the polymorphism of apo-E as it relates to plasma lipoprotein metabolism may prove to be a major contributor to CAD risk in the general population.

Apo-E can occur as one of three proteins called "isoforms," which result from a gene containing one of three specific apo-E alleles. Each apo-E can be isolated by isoelectric focusing. Alleles apo-e_2, apo-e_3, and apo-e_4 can provide the following isoform patterns: E_2E_2, E_2E_3, E_3E_3, E_3E_4, or E_4E_4. Apo-E_2 represents the abnormal gene product and occurs in 10 percent of the population. The abnormality associated with familial dysbetalipoproteinemia occurs with the homozygotic E_2E_2 condition, which, although present in five percent of the population, causes a clinical disorder in only one in 10,000 individuals. The underlying apo-E isoform appears to have a structural change due to a reduction in positive charge resulting from an amino acid base substitution. This mutant apo-E has a decreased LDL-C receptor affinity that slows VLDL-C/LDL-C metabolism, resulting in plasma accumulation of the remnant IDL-C or broad band (VLDL-remnant) particle.

Because apo-E modulates the metabolism of apo-B-containing lipoproteins, it can influence the plasma cholesterol and triglyceride levels in the general population. The apo-E_2E_2 isoform, which is poorly taken up by cell receptors, causes less intercellular cholesterol uptake resulting in upregulation of the LDL (apo-B, -E) receptor. Plasma triglyceride levels are elevated and plasma cholesterol levels are depressed in this setting (Type III), while the converse occurs in the apo-E_4E_4 setting. Apo-E polymorphism may have a major role in influencing CAD risk in the general population.

Lipoprotein (a)

Apo "little a" [Lp(a)] continues to achieve increasing recognition for its role in CAD risk. This could be considered as an autosomal dominant disorder; familial hyper Lp (a), which is observed in 30 percent of members of families with a premature history of CAD. The relationship of apo (a) to CAD risk may stem from its structural resemblance to plasminogen (thrombogenesis) as well as to LDL (atherogenesis). Lp (a) is synthesized hepatically by LDL-independent routes and constitutes an LDL-like particle (density = 1.05 to 1.10 g/ml). Lp (a) contains a specific glycoprotein linked to apo-B by disulfide bonds. It has been suggested that Lp (a) may block fibrinolytic activity because of its resemblance to plasmin ogen and may contribute to the thromboatherogenic process. Plasma Lp (a) level directly reflects family history of CAD and has a suggested potential role in clinical practice for identification of the genetically high-risk patient. Alternatively, recent findings from the Helsinky Heart Study fail to demonstrate that Lp(a) levels were predictive of CAD risk. Currently, no known dietary or pharmaceutical approaches are available to lower Lp (a) levels, although preliminary evidence suggests niacin may be effective.

Cholesteryl Ester Transfer Protein (CETP)

Although not technically classified as an apolipoprotein, CETP plays an important role in lipid metabolism. Shown in Figure 4.3 CETP participates in the reverse cholesterol transport by exchanging equimolar concentrations of cholesteryl esters from HDL to VLDL and LDL in exchange for triglycerides (see Figure 4.3). Thus, cholesteryl ester clearance is increased through the VLDL/LDC particle system, which could promote atherosclerosis. Plasma HDL-C level is inversely related to CETP activity. The relationship of CETP activity to CAD risk is uncertain. It is suggested that individuals with Familial CETP deficiency (an autosomal dominant disorder) have a reduced CAD risk, particularly because of their increased levels of HDL-C. This condition is described as a cause of familial hyperalphalipoproteinemia, known as "the longevity syndrome".

References

Carlson LA, Hamsten A, Asplund A: Pronounced lowering of serum levels of lipoprotein Lp (a) in hyperlipidaemic subjects treated with nicotinic acid. J Intern Med 1989;226:271.

Currington PN, Hunt L, Ishola M, et al: Apolipoproteins (a), A1 and parental history in men with early onset of ischaemic heart disease. Lancet 1988; 1:1070.

Davignon J, Gregg RE, et al: Apolipoprotein E polymorphism atherosclerosis. Arteriosclerosis 1988;8:1.

Editorial: 'Lp (a)' joins other serum cholesterol lipoproteins as a risk determinant. JAMA 1989; 261:2013.

Grundy SM, Chait A, Runzell JD: Familial combined hyperlipidemia workshop. Arteriosclerosis 1987;7:203.

Hoefler G, Harnoncourt F, Paschke E, et al: Lipoprotein (a), a risk factor for myocardial infarction. Arteriosclerosis 1988;8:398.

Javhiainen M, Koskinen P, Ehnholm C, et al: Lipoprotein (a) and coronary heart disease risk: a rested control study of the Helsinky Heart Study participants. Atherosclerosis 1991;89:59.

Kissebah AH, Alfarsi S, Evans DJ: Low density lipoprotein metabolism in familial combined hyperlipidemia. Arteriosclerosis 1984;4:614.

Kottke BA, Moll PP, Michels VV, Weidman WH: Levels of lipids, lipoproteins and apolipoproteins in a defined population. Mayo Clin Proc 1991;66:1198.

Li W-H, Tanimura M, Luo C-C, et al: The apolipoprotein multigene family: biosynthesis, structure-function relationships and evolution. J Lipid Res 1988;29:245.

McPherson R, Mann CJ, Tall AR, et al: Plasma concentrations of CETP in hyperlipoproteinemia. Athero and Throm. 1991;11:797.

Naito HK: The clinical significance of apolipoprotein measurements. J Clin Immun 1986;9:11.

Stampfer MJ, Sacks FM, Salvini S, et al: A prospective study of cholesterol, apolipoproteins and the risk of myocardial infarction. N Engl J Med 1991;325:373.

Uterman G: The mysteries of lipoprotein (a). Science 1989;246:904.

Yamashita S, Hui DY, Wetterav JR, et al: Characterization of plasma lipoproteins in patients with CETP deficiency. Metabolism 1991;40:756.